"This book is the valuable contribution of psychoanalysts from different regions who have developed ideas and hypotheses about the vicissitudes of pregnancy in cases of infertility and reproductive techniques. The different chapters written by psychoanalysts with vast experience in this field contribute with their understanding and ideas to the various types of problems that come to our consulting rooms nowadays."

Patricia Alkolombre, *Argentinean Psychoanalytic Association, COWAP Overall-Chair*

"This book is leading the way for psychoanalysis in contemporary times, moving psychoanalysts and psychotherapists into today's world. The editors have collected contributions from diverse regions bringing thoughtful and refreshing considerations on infertility, surrogacy and donors, the passion for a child, along with pregnancy and pregnancy losses. Exploration of origin and birth fantasies, surrogacy clinic consultation, along with regional cultural mythology, offer the reader a textured innovative immersion on psychoanalytic thinking in the current times of reproduction technologies."

Paula Ellman, *Ph.D., Contemporary Freudian Society, Former COWAP Overall-Chair*

"This book is a stroke of luck in several respects: the clinically and theoretically highly qualified, often emotionally moving contributions by all the authors from different countries around the world not only enable a deeper understanding of the feelings associated with the desire to have children, pregnancy, infertility and assisted reproduction, as well as the associated help for all those affected. Instead of focusing on deficits, the authors place the psychological development of parenthood at the center of their work. This includes working with the possibilities of assisted reproduction, and not against them – remaining at the same time open to the complexity of unconscious connections and conflicts. This shows how lively psychoanalysis can be in the 21st century."

Heribert Blass, *Dr. med., German Psychoanalytic Association, IPA President-elect*

T0383432

Pregnancy, Assisted Reproduction, and Psychoanalysis

Pregnancy, Assisted Reproduction, and Psychoanalysis reflects on contemporary views on pregnancy, while offering guidance on how to work with women and couples experiencing infertility as well as the unique issues raised by having a child through assisted reproduction technologies.

Comprised of chapters written by eminent analysts working with infertile couples and women, and parents who have a child born from assisted reproduction, this book offers insightful ways to better understand the challenges these patients undertake and the various issues this might bring into the analytic room. The contributors examine the myriad psychic problems subjects are confronted with which could impact their ability to bond with children born through ART: the mourning processes infertility entails, the identification with the fertile parental couple, the unconscious representation of origin, the representation of the primal scene, and the process of symbolic affiliation. They consider the working-through these processes necessitate in order to enable filiation and healthy parenting, and give invaluable tools to the analyst to enable the promotion of psychological growth. Throughout, the chapters address the emotions that infertility summons in which both patient and analyst find a spectrum of unconscious phantasies and anxieties.

This book is an essential read for psychoanalysts and other professionals working in the field of ART, as well as those interested in motherhood and its vicissitudes and intersection with psychoanalysis.

Renata Viola Vives is a psychoanalyst for children, adolescents, and adults and a COWAP Latin-American representative. She has worked in the field of assisted reproduction for 15 years.

Ana Teresa Vale is a clinical psychologist and psychoanalyst living and working in Lisbon. Currently COWAP European representative, she is also part of the editorial board of the *Portuguese Psychoanalytic Journal*.

Psychoanalysis and Women Series
Series Editor: Paula Ellman

Myths of Mighty Women
Their Application in Psychoanalytic Psychotherapy
Edited by Arlene Kramer Richards, Lucille Spira

Medea
Myth and Unconscious Fantasy
Edited by Esa Roos

The Status of Women
Violence, Identity, and Activism
Edited by Vivian B. Pender

Changing Sexualities and Parental Functions in the Twenty-First Century
Changing Sexualities, Changing Parental Functions
Cândida Sé Holovko, Frances Thomson-Salo

The Courage to Fight Violence Against Women
Psychoanalytic and Multidisciplinary Perspectives
Edited by Paula L. Ellman, Nancy R. Goodman

When a Child is Abused
Towards Psychoanalytic Understanding and Therapy
Edited by Frances Thompson-Salo, Laura Tognoli Pasquali

Pregnancy, Assisted Reproduction, and Psychoanalysis
Renata Viola Vives, Ana Teresa Vale

For more information about this series, please visit: https://www.routledge.com/Psychoanalysis-and-Women-Series/book-series/KARNACPWS

Pregnancy, Assisted Reproduction, and Psychoanalysis

Edited by Renata Viola Vives and Ana Teresa Vale

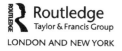
Routledge
Taylor & Francis Group

LONDON AND NEW YORK

Designed cover image: ©Getty

First published 2025
by Routledge
4 Park Square, Milton Park, Abingdon, Oxon OX14 4RN

and by Routledge
605 Third Avenue, New York, NY 10158

Routledge is an imprint of the Taylor & Francis Group, an informa business

British Library Cataloguing-in-Publication Data
A catalogue record for this book is available from the British Library

ISBN: 978-1-032-69343-9 (hbk)
ISBN: 978-1-032-63982-6 (pbk)
ISBN: 978-1-032-69344-6 (ebk)

DOI: 10.4324/9781032693446

Typeset in Times New Roman
by SPi Technologies India Pvt Ltd (Straive)

Contents

Editors

Renata Viola Vives is a clinical psychologist and psychoanalyst who lives and works in Porto Alegre, Brazil. She is a full member of the Brazilian Society of Psychoanalysis in Porto Alegre, where she has been coordinating a study group on assisted reproduction since 2012. She has been a part of COWAP since 2018, being a liaison member of her Society. She is a member of the COWAP Brasil Commission, where she organizes scientific events and edits COWAP Brasil books. Currently, she is a Latin-American representative of the Committee and, as such, has participated in the organization of COWAP conferences, and worked in the organization of COWAP panels in IPA, Fepal and Febrapsi meetings, as well as other institutions. She regularly participates in international psychoanalytic events, where she has already presented several scientific works. Several of her articles have been published in different psychoanalytic books and journals. She is an editor and organizer of books on parenting, assisted reproduction, and adoption (*Essays on Assisted Reproduction, Parenting and Adoption*, volume 1 and 2 and *Psychoanalytic Reflections on Assisted Reproduction*, published in Portuguese in 2021 and 2022, by Gênese Editora). She has scientific researches on the topic of assisted reproduction, also documented in scientific papers.

Ana Teresa Vale is a clinical psychologist and a psychoanalyst living and working in Lisbon, Portugal. She is a full member of the Portuguese Psychoanalytic Society, teaching in her society's training program. She is currently part of the editorial board of the *Portuguese Psychoanalytic Journal*. She has been part of COWAP since 2012, having started as the liaison member of the Portuguese Society. She is now a European representative of the Committee, and as such she has facilitated study groups on infertility and assisted reproduction, has participated in the organization of international COWAP conferences and has worked on COWAP panel organizations in the EPF and IPA meetings. She participates regularly in international psychoanalytic events, where she has on several occasions presented her work. Several of her papers have been published in different languages in books and psychoanalytic journals.

Contributors

Conceição Tavares de Almeida is a clinical psychologist and training and supervising member of the Portuguese Psychoanalytical Society, also a child and adolescent psychoanalyst. She was an IPA Board Member (European representative elected for 2021–2023), part of the Appointments Committee, of the ad hoc working group on prejudice, discrimination, and racism, and functioned as a link between the IPA Board and the European Societies. She is currently the president of the Portuguese Psychoanalytical Society. In the past, she was chair of the Education Committee (2022–2024), vice-president (2015–2019) and scientific secretary (2011–2015). She was also a COWAP liaison member from 2015 to 2023 and a member of the Scientific Committee of the *Portuguese Journal of Psychoanalysis* and the French journal *Cliniques*. She is the published author of several papers and co-author of national and international books.

Christine Anzieu-Premmereur is a psychiatrist and psychoanalyst in New York City, who works in private practice with adults, children, parents and their babies. A member of the Société Psychanalytique de Paris (Paris Psychoanalytic Society), she is on the faculty of the Columbia Psychoanalytic Center for Training and Research and she is an Assistant Clinical Professor in Psychiatry at Columbia University. She is the chair of the IPA Committee for Child and Adolescent Psychoanalysis (COCAP). She recently published "The process of representation in early childhood" (2013) and "Attacks on linking in parents of young disturbed children" (2017). She co-edited with Vaia Tsolas *A psychoanalytic exploration of the body in today's world* (Routledge, 2017) and *A psychoanalytic exploration of the contemporary search for pleasure: The turning of the screw* (Routledge, 2024).

Sofía Barandiaran Pérez-Yarza is an associate member of the APM (Madrid Psychoanalytical Association). She started her training with a PGDip in psychoanalytic observational studies at the Tavistock Clinic. She has been working in private practice with children, adolescents, and adults since 2002. In recent years, she has given a series of lectures on the taboos surrounding motherhood, which have been summarized in the article: "The Taboo of Motherhood" (*APM Journal*, 2022). She has also lectured on infancy, adolescence and on topics such as "The masculine, in crisis?", a paper shortly to be published.

Katy Bogliatto is a child psychiatrist and training analyst of the Belgian Psychoanalytical Society, liaison member for the Committee of Children and Adolescent Psychoanalysis (COCAP), and vice-president elect of the International Psychoanalytical Association (2023–2025). She teaches at the Free University of Brussels, third cycle on the Certificate in Children & Adolescent Psychotherapeutic Clinic and on The Training in Clinical Psychology of Family and Couple Diversity. She also teaches at GECFAPPE (Early childhood psychoanalytic family therapy). She's member of the editorial board of the *Revue Belge de Psychanalyse*. She works in private practice with adults, adolescents, children, and young toddlers (parenthood-centered psychotherapy) and at the Assisted Reproduction Center of Chirec, Brussels.

Graciela Cardó Soria is a clinical psychologist and a full member of the Peruvian Society of Psychoanalysis (SPP), of which she is currently president. She is professor of the Graduate School of the Pontifical Catholic University of Peru and of the Institute of the Peruvian Society of Psychoanalysis. She has been part of COWAP since 2005, and started as liaison member of the Peruvian Society of Psychoanalysis in 2012. She is currently the COWAP Co-Chair for Latin America. She has organized the XV Intergenerational Latin American Dialogue titled "Women, gender, culture, future" and has participated in multiple IPA, FEPAL, and COWAP meetings as a speaker. She is co-editor of the books *Masculino-Femenino: Diversidad, Género, Transformaciones* (2019), *Mariam Alizade. Ideas Centrales a la Luz de la Crisis Actual* (2022), and *Poder, Género y Amor* (2022).

Eleonora Di Lucia is a psychoanalytic psychotherapist of children, adolescents, and couples. Member of the SIPsIA (Società Italiana di Psicoterapia Psicoanalitica del Bambino, dell'Adolescente e della Coppia). Working with children, adolescents, and parents both in private practice and at the social cooperative *Nostos* and the clinical centre "Tana libera tutti" of the SIPsIA. Author of articles for the journal *Richard & Piggle*. Founding member of the organisation *PMA – Ponte per una Maternità Attesa*.

Veronika Garms is a psychoanalytic psychotherapist of children, adolescents, and couples. Ordinary member of the SIPsIA (Società Italiana di Psicoterapia Psicoanalitica del Bambino, dell'Adolescente e della Coppia). Delegate of the SIPsIA and the Winnicott Institute at the European Federation of Psychoanalytic Psychotherapy (EFPP). Member of the editorial board of *Richard & Piggle*, a psychoanalytic journal for infancy and adolescence. Author of articles published in the journals *Kinderanalyse* and *Richard & Piggle*. Co-editor of the book *La teoria dei processi maturativi di Winnicott* (2022). Founding member of the organisation *PMA – Ponte per una Maternità Attesa*.

Selene Mancinelli is a psychoanalytic psychotherapist of children, adolescents, and couples. Member of the SIPsIA (Società Italiana di Psicoterapia Psicoanalitica del Bambino, dell'Adolescente e della Coppia). Working with children, adolescents and parents both in private practice and at the two clinical centers, "Sanem Somalia" and "Tana Libera Tutti", of the SIPsIA. Author of articles for the journal *Richard & Piggle*. Founding member of the organisation *PMA – Ponte per una Maternità Attesa*.

Paola Marion has a PhD in philosophy, is a training and supervising analyst for the Italian Psychoanalytic Society, and a child and adolescent psychoanalyst. She is past chair of the IPA Outreach Committee for Europe (2009–2011) and past editor of the *Rivista Italiana di Psicoanalisi* (2017–2021). She has been a member of the European Group Exploring Training Process and Practice (ETPP). Her main study and research interests concern the topic of sexuality in psychoanalysis, the question of *Nachträglichkeit*, the transmission of psychoanalysis. She has published papers in the *International Journal of Psychoanalysis* and in other journals, and presented papers at the IPA and EPF congresses. Her book, *Il disagio del desiderio. Sessualità e fecondazione al tempo delle biotecnologie*, published in 2017, has been translated into English and published by Routledge in 2021 with the title *Sexuality and procreation at the age of biotechnology. Desire and its discontents*.

Giovanna Pavanello is a psychoanalytic psychotherapist of children, adolescents, and couples. Member of the SIPsIA (Società Italiana di Psicoterapia Psicoanalitica del Bambino, dell'Adolescente e della Coppia). Working with children, adolescents and parents both in private practice and at the clinical centre "Tana Libera Tutti" within the SIPsIA. Since 2019, member of the Management Committee at the clinical center "Tana Libera Tutti". Curator of the Italian digitalisation of *Edoardo Weiss Archive*. Author of the paper "Edoardo Weiss" for *Appendice VIII della Enciclopedia Italiana di Scienze, Lettere ed Arti* (edited by Istituto della Enciclopedia Italiana founded by Giovanni Treccani). Founding member of the organisation *PMA – Ponte per una Maternità Attesa*.

Emanuela Quagliata is a psychoanalyst and child and adolescent psychoanalyst of the Italian Psychoanalytic Society and child, adolescent and family psychoanalytic psychotherapist trained at the Tavistock Clinic (ACP). She is currently COWAP Co-Chair for Europe and Consultant in the IPA Committee on Child and Adolescent Psychoanalysis (COCAP). She wrote her doctorate dissertation on "Psychoanalytic perspective on recurrent miscarriage and autoimmune disease". She has written widely on child analysis, child development, and eating disorders, amongst which: *Becoming parents and overcoming obstacles: A psychoanalytic perspective on miscarriage, premature birth, infertility and post-natal depression* (Karnac, 2013); *101bambino* (www.101bambino.com) (Astrolabio-Routledge) and *An introduction on child analysis* (Routledge, 2024).

Nancy Tame Ayub is a *clinical psychologist*, with training in family and couples therapy and a doctoral intern in psychotherapy at the Mexican Psychoanalytic Association (APM), living and working in Mexico City. She is a training psychoanalyst at the Mexican Psychoanalytic Association, teaches seminars at the Institute of Psychoanalysis, and is on the Library Committee of her association. She is the author of two books on the emotional aspects of infertility: *Infertility. An Accompanying Guide in the Search for a New Being* (2016, published in Spanish) and *Infertility. The Secret Pain Methods to Reverse It* (2007, published in Spanish). The process and the emotional impact experienced by people facing reproductive problems is one of the main subjects in the papers she has presented during her career, in the articles she has published in magazines, and in the chapters for books she has written on this topic. The interest in providing information about the myth of psychogenic infertility and the risks of working with this belief is a constant commitment in her clinical and academic work.

Melis Tanik Sivri, PsyD is a founding member, current vice-president and a training and supervising analyst of Psike Istanbul. She is a COWAP European representative and the COWAP liaison member of Psike Istanbul. She is the editor-in-chief of the annuals of the *International Journal of Psychoanalysis (IJP)* and former editor of the *Turkish Annual* of the *IJP*. She has various translations and publications on femininity, motherhood, pregnancy, and assisted reproductive techniques as well as women artists, in Turkish and English. The books she edited and co-edited are *Women Analyzing Women* (with E. Abrevaya, 2020); *Reflective Affinities* (with C. Joannidis, 2013); *The "Other" Side of Psychoanalysis: Heinz Kohut* (with Y. Erten & N. Mitrani, 2004). She was the recipient of the 2011 Psychoanalytic Writings Award given by the Istanbul Psychoanalytical Association with her article "Frida Kahlo: The Silent Scream Transmitted from Mirror to Canvas". She translated "Introduction to the Work of Melanie Klein" by Hanna Segal into Turkish (2023).

Foreword

Patricia Alkolombre

It is my pleasure, as the Overall Chair of the Committee on Women and Psychoanalysis (COWAP) of the International Psychoanalytic Association, to write the foreword to this book *Pregnancy, Assisted Reproduction, and Psychoanalysis*, compiled by Renata Viola Vives (COWAP Latin America representative member) and Ana Teresa Vale (COWAP Europe representative member). This valuable work consists of contemporary conceptions regarding the vicissitudes of pregnancy, infertility and assisted reproductive techniques (ART) from both the clinical and the theoretical points of view. This publication is a part of the growing series of COWAP books on psychoanalysis and women.

COWAP was established in 1998 by Otto Kernberg during his presidency. The project was created by Joan Raphael-Leff in order to promote the development of the gender perspective in theoretical and clinical psychoanalysis and to explore women's issues. The creation of COWAP, a committee led by women, was innovative at the IPA, since at that point most of the psychoanalysts in charge were men. By that time, dialogues between psychoanalysis and gender studies had already begun to develop, initially around femininity and women's issues.

At the first COWAP meeting, Joan Raphael-Leff (EU), Helen Meyers (NA), Beth Seelig (NA), and Mariam Alizade (LA) defined the basis of the relationship between COWAP members through a fraternal spirit and an active participation of different generations of analysts, both members and candidates.

COWAP's proposal was to provide a framework for the exploration of topics relating to issues primarily of concern to women. In 2001, under the presidency of Mariam Alizade (2001–2005), the themes were expanded to include issues related to men and their relationship to women, gender-related topics, and how culture plays a role in the development of theories. COWAP conducted research on problems concerning the complex relations between categories of psychoanalysis, sexuality, and gender. Otto Kernberg, in his speech addressed in the first COWAP Conference in Buenos Aires, in May 1999 said:

The mutual fertilization between psychoanalytic theory and contemporary feminist analysis has advanced our understanding of the relationships between normal and pathological development on the one hand, and the impact of cultural and ideological changes on the other.

As can be seen, the exchange through theoretical-clinical discussions on topics of social relevance was made within an interdisciplinary framework from the outset. Since its foundation, COWAP aims to constantly maintain an open space for reflection, questioning, and exchange with other disciplines on complex issues such as femininity, masculinity, women's and men's issues, hierarchical gender relations, gender-based violence, and parenthood and reproductive techniques.

This book includes the contributions of valuable psychoanalysts from different regions who have developed ideas and hypotheses about the vicissitudes of pregnancy in cases of infertility and assisted reproductive techniques. Throughout the chapters, the authors display scenarios in which the psychic and relational aspects intertwine with medical studies and diagnostics related to infertility. It is clear throughout the book that ART procedures demand that patients and analysts work through the vicissitudes of infertility and the emotional impact it has, either in the couple or the ART–born child.

The phantasmatic and the ominous aspects that may be present in these parenting projects are discussed together with their repercussions on children born through ART. The parent-child bond is also analyzed within this clinical context. Mourning and grief take part in this particular journey, both in individual or couple consultations: the representations and fantasies about the origins of the children together with the primal scene, among other topics, are discussed in this book.

Lastly, the different chapters, written by psychoanalysts with vast experience in this field, contribute with their understanding and ideas to the various types of problems that come into our consulting rooms nowadays.

Preface

The *Women and Psychoanalysis Book Series* grew from the work of the International Psychoanalytical Association Committee on Women and Psychoanalysis (COWAP). The IPA-Routledge series furthers global perspectives and creativities on topics related to women, gender and sexuality and psychoanalysis, including intersections with diversity and cross-cultural experience.

With the increasingly rapid advances in reproductive technologies and the arenas to which they give rise, *Pregnancy, Assisted Reproduction, and Psychoanalysis*, co-edited by Renata Viola Vives (Brazil) and Ana Teresa Vale (Portugal), offers an in-depth psychoanalytic approach to the field of reproductive technologies and the intensely personal and psychological issues to which they give rise. This area has often been limited by a tendency to pathologize, to approach infertility as the result of psychic conflict and to dismiss those who begin the difficult processes involved as omnipotent or in denial. The breadth of voices gathered in this volume demonstrates the complexity of psychic difficulty encountered and the need to investigate them carefully and without prejudice.

Alternative family constellations, forms of motherhood, and conceptions of femininity and the accompanying expansion of new subjectivities potentially challenge both the foundational tenets of psychoanalysis and the normative assumptions to which they sometimes give rise. This book offers a series of studies addressing specific clinical problems, the psychoanalysis of an infertile woman, the intervention in a family that carries the secret of ART and its effects on the child's development, the psychic challenges for the donor and the understanding of taboos around donation, a patient's representation of pregnancy and loss, an account of surrogacy and its links with maternal preoccupation, and consultations at a governmental ART clinic. There are chapters that consider cinematic and social media representations of the continuing psychic complexities of all forms of reproduction. We are proud to publish this volume by Vives and Vale in our series as a model of psychoanalytic thinking in the contemporary world.

The *Women and Psychoanalysis Book Series* Editorial Board represents all regions of the IPA, with six editors collaborating as a team from Goa, London, Lima, Milan, San Francisco, and Washington DC. We are women editors and writers active in psychoanalysis regionally and in the IPA. We encourage single author and multiple author book proposal submissions on topics of women, gender, femininity, and masculinity in the consulting room and in the wider world of culture and history. The Board offers consultation and guidance in the crafting of proposals and throughout the writing and publishing process.

The Women and Psychoanalysis Book Series Editorial Board
Paula Ellman (Editor-in-Chief)
Carolina Bacchi
Sara Boffito
Lesley Caldwell
Paula Escribens Pareja
Amrita Narayanan

Chapter 1

Introduction

Renata Viola Vives and Ana Teresa Vale

The book *Pregnancy, Assisted Reproduction, and Psychoanalysis* was conceived in our minds during the years that we have been working in the field of assisted reproduction (AR) and its psychological vicissitudes. But it is the encounters between bodies and subjectivities that transform the imaginary baby into a real baby, and it was the encounter provided by COWAP, which brought together colleagues from all over the world who are interested in these themes, which shaped this book that the reader holds right now.

This publication was born out of the need to make accessible all the work that COWAP colleagues have been doing, which has often gone somewhat invisible in the psychoanalytic community as a whole. Despite the fact that AR is an increasingly present topic in our clinical practice, myths and prejudices remain rooted that can prevent a therapeutic or analytical work from being fruitful.

Incidentally, the relationship between psychoanalysis and AR has been somewhat troubled, given that older authors tended to consider infertility, pregnancy loss, and other reproductive upheavals as exclusively resulting from women's unconscious intrapsychic conflicts. This interpretation ended up being accusatory, reducing infertility to the idea that, if a woman does not get pregnant, it is because she does not want the baby.

Furthermore, when AR techniques began to develop, they were sometimes considered by analysts to be omnipotent movements, and therefore pathological ones, with the idea being disseminated that, for a woman suffering from infertility, the "healthy" way out of it would be to mourn her fertility and accept the idea of a life without biological children.

Thus conveying an idealization of the feminine, which only materializes through motherhood, and an idealization of motherhood, the one that counts being the one that happens "naturally", and in which the mother sacrifices herself for her baby and is always attentive to the needs of her children, to the detriment of her own needs, psychoanalytic theory has kept many women and couples away from analysts' offices. Therefore, these people went looking for other ways to deal with their psychological suffering resulting from infertility and the treatments they are subjected to (Leon, 1996).

DOI: 10.4324/9781032693446-1

With this publication, we want to highlight the various problems and questions that AR may bring, but we also want to show that there are many forms of motherhood and many feminine identities. The female identity, like the psychic construction of the role of the mother, is an idiosyncratic construction, based on a multiplicity of early and later experiences; primary and secondary unconscious identifications, anxieties, and fantasies; unconscious representations of different natures. For this reason, there are as many feminine identities as there are women; there are as many motherhoods as there are mothers.

And in fact, in recent decades, we have experienced constant changes in our society, which have brought new subjectivities, as well as new models of parenting and family, which call into question our theories and psychoanalytic framework. The concepts of origin, primal scene, and oedipal configuration, which will be discussed in the chapters of this book, are put into question and ask for further theoretical developments as babies are born out of surrogacy or through AR procedures that involve much more than just mommy and daddy. In fact, all these technological and social changes give rise to new family structures where different people play roles that didn't exist in the traditional family, necessarily influencing the emotional and sexual development of the child.

Among these changes, the issue of motherhood has been undergoing constant transformations. From the 1960s onward, with the advent of sexual liberation and contraception, in the Western world motherhood was no longer seen as a destiny, as a woman's duty. Abortion became legal in several countries, although today there is still a lot of discrepancy around the world in relation to this issue. Chatel (1995) also recalls the impact that contraception had, separating the sexual act from procreation, making the idea of a child increasingly distant from the idea of sex.

These changes brought the child more as an object of the woman's conscious wish, together with the unconscious desire, where safe contraception would temporarily sterilize her and a conscious decision would release her again for fertility. Thus making the woman believe that she controlled her fertility by being able to inhibit it, becoming responsible for everything that happened to her, for being the inhabitant of the body capable of gestating, which altered the relationship of women with their female body and with their sexuality.

Resulting from these changes, the popular concepts of women, motherhood, and femininity are being reinvented in our societies. At the same time that the birth rate has decreased in Western countries, the age (on average) of first pregnancy has been postponed, and sterility has become voluntary.

Nonetheless, at the same proportion that reproduction tended to become voluntary, cases of infertility grew. According to the WHO, with data from April 2023, 1 in 6 people worldwide are affected by infertility at some point in their lives, and a couple is considered infertile after a year of trying to get pregnant without using contraceptives methods, not differing much in high-, middle-, and low-income countries (Keenan, 2023). Infertility is often unconsciously associated with disability and worthlessness in women, while in men it is often equated with impotence.

In this same context, reproductive technologies emerged, which brought about significant changes by intervening at the bodily level. Artificial insemination and the different *in vitro* fertilization techniques, to some extent, have remedied infertility, allowing a pregnancy. In the late 1970s, in England, the first baby was born after being conceived in a test tube. Since then, more than ten million children have been born in the world using assisted human reproduction techniques, according to SBRA data (Queiroz, 2023).

Assisted reproduction, a term that designates a series of methods and techniques that make it possible to carry out pregnancies that would not happen spontaneously, that is, that place medical-technological intervention as a condition for its occurrence, has been shown to be a modern and widely disseminated approach to address childlessness (Ramirez-Galvez, 2007).

If beforehand we did not face doubts about what it is to be a mother, we are currently facing countless uncertainties. Genetic studies gave us certainty about who the biological parent is, but not necessarily who will carry out maternal and paternal functions. As such, AR technologies challenge our certainties, redefining the concepts of maternity, paternity, and filiation, at the conscious and unconscious level.

Assisted fertilization with own gametes or donated gametes, the freezing of eggs or embryos, the surplus embryos, and the surrogate pregnancy are some of the medical solutions to infertility. Medicine continues to add new solutions, some of them sounding like something out of science fiction movies.

In fact, the intervention of biotechnology, which initially focused on infertility, has extended to many other situations, among which are the postponement of motherhood in situations of prolonged illness, in situations linked to the professional life (especially for women), in situations of absence of a partner or limitations related to age, as well as parenting projects for homosexual couples, which are no longer reduced to adoption.

The desire for a child, from the first attempts at conception until birth, is always permeated by anxieties and unconscious fantasies. These fantasies begin to be built in the earliest childhood of both the boy and the girl, are subject to transformation as the child grows and develops, and later on will be revisited when forming a couple. These anxieties and fantasies will also need to be negotiated and worked through in the transition to parenthood.

However, when facing infertility, women and couples will face different challenges. We can find different scenarios, all coming with consequences for the emotional well-being of all parties involved – undiagnosed situations that force couples to face and live with uncertainty, unsuccessful treatments and pregnancy losses that demand a very difficult work of mourning, gamete donation or embryo adoption that come with the need to elaborate the presence of another party and all the fantasies that it entails, surrogacy that brings to the scene another body (and another mind). All these situations that AR brings to the lives of contemporary patients demand a deep reflection and empathy from the part of the clinician.

Assisted reproduction procedures may function as a third party in this relationship in the sense that, instead of a sexual encounter, parents and children will have to deal with a scene or a set of technological scenes, medical exams, procedures, and medical staff, as well as donors and recipients (in many cases) and a series of fantasies and anxieties that do not belong to the universe of so-called "natural" reproduction; and all this after many wounds experienced by infertility.

In psychoanalysis, the first works on infertility come from Helene Deutsch (1960), followed by the work of Dinora Pines (1972) and Marie Langer (1981).

Helene Deutsch believed that women who were more immature tended to put themselves in a fragile and dependent position. In her perspective, these women were not able to step up to an adult position, which is why they ended up incapable of conceiving.

In Deutsch's opinion, in infertile women, paranoid fears prevail, which is why the woman would build different barriers against the incorporation of the penis and semen or against sheltering the fetus, where the most superficial barrier may be the fear of defloration. In this context, frigidity could be a defense, as well as hormonal disorders, which would lead to the temporary damage to her femininity. When facing infertility, often the main interest of their lives would then become the infertility treatments.

For Marie Langer (1981), on the other hand, her starting point was the study of women who could not get pregnant, but who from a physical point of view did not present any problem (at least, problems detectable by the medicine of the time). Langer stated that, when these women were facing the possibility of realizing their conscious desires, they became so anxious that they could lose, albeit temporarily, their fertility. She then deduced that their unconscious conflict with motherhood would have influenced their choice of partner and would later disturb their possibility of conceiving or carrying out a pregnancy. In her view, the unconscious conflict itself would come from early frustrations in a phase of extreme dependence in the relationship to the mother.

For her part, Pines (1972) placed these problems in the context of the processes of elaboration linked to the different phases of a woman's development, namely the processes of psychic separation from her mother, and highlighted the presence of intense ambivalence, conflicts, and early traumas in cases of women with recurrent pregnancy losses and/or fertility problems.

Although these authors' ideas may be interesting, they are not applicable to all women and couples in these situations. On the other hand, they are still a simplistic approach to a very complex problem, conveying an omnipotent idea of psychoanalysis – in their work, reproductive problems were solved with analysis.

On the contrary, today we know that the work of analysis in these cases is not solving infertility in a direct and literal sense, but helping the woman to work out all the suffering and psychic consequences that this situation can bring. Furthermore, AR procedures open up new possibilities that didn't exist in the second half of the 20th century, when these authors wrote their work. Naturally, they didn't contemplate all the complexity of the situations we find nowadays.

Along these lines, it is worth remembering the work of Sylvie Faure-Pragier (2003, 2008), who argues that we cannot conceive a direct and linear causality for infertility or for reproductive problems in general. In her opinion, the label "psychogenic infertility" is meaningless.

Faure-Pragier proposes a psychosomatic understanding of any infertility situation, in which unconscious aspects always play a role. But in her perspective, it's not only in sterility without a medical cause that emotional aspects take place – these play a fundamental role in any reproductive project. In fact, the author herself speaks of the psychosomatic nature of reproduction, in which the psyche uses the body as an intermediary for the expression of its unconscious conflicts, fantasies, and emotions.

Several other authors (Alkolombre, 2008, 2023; Raphael-Leff, 2013; Mann, 2014; Ansermet, 2017; Vives, 2021, 2022; Marion, 2022) are currently helping us to rethink these older ideas, offering new meanings to infertility and to the conundrums patients face when they turn to AR. Many authors within psychoanalysis, some of whom are part of this book, have addressed these issues exploring different aspects of this very complex problem, and the focus has shifted from the etiological aspect itself to the psychic consequences that these situations entail.

Therefore, this book aims at thinking on the contemporary world and its promises regarding pregnancy, infertility, and AR, examining new psychic problems subjects are confronted with, which will need elaboration and working-through, in order to enable filiation and parenthood and allow growth. Either working with the infertile couple / woman or with the AR–born child, in this book psychoanalysts look for ways of better understanding the challenges the patients undertake, and what kind of problems this brings into the analytic room.

We open the book with the theme of origins and secrecy with "Fantasies of origin and the origin of fantasies." Paola Marion and collaborators suggest that the secrecy about the intervention of AR in the birth of children reveals the parents' difficulty in metabolizing not only the infertility that led them to AR procedures, but also the physical and psychical suffering that was involved in such births. Using clinical vignettes, the authors also explore the challenges children and analysts may face while working through the child's primitive fantasies.

For her part, Emanuela Quagliata, in "Illusion, illusional belief and mourning in infertility," seeks to deepen the understanding of the unconscious dynamics of a group of patients who, while asking for help in relation to their psychological suffering linked to the difficulty in getting pregnant, then show themselves very resistant to the analytic work and relationship. Focusing on clinical material, it is suggested that this happens because the analytic process forces them to question deeply unconsciously invested convictions and demand mourning processes that these patients find very difficult.

Melis Tanik Sivri writes about feelings of envy, shame and shaming in the face of infertility based on the Turkish movie "The Empty Cradle" in a chapter titled after the movie. She explores how these feelings of envy and shame are constituted in women through the character of Fatma and how women who have difficulty conceiving end up having intense feelings of idealization, envy, and competition towards other women who they consider fertile.

The story of Pinocchio, the film "Artificial Intelligence," and some examples from social media serve Graciela Cardó in her chapter "Reflections on the concept of 'Passion for a Child'," to address the concept of Passion for a Child, described by Alkolombre in 2008. In this chapter, the author works with the triad of passion, alienation, and idealization.

Nancy Tame Ayub focuses her chapter titled "Emotional aspects of donors" on the psyche of donors. When we talk about gamete donation, we usually think about the people who receive these donations and the psychic consequences of needing to resort to this type of procedure. However, we rarely address the donors' motivations and the potential après-coup that this decision may have later on, which may take on new and unexpected meanings, requiring elaboration and working-through.

In her chapter "Live babies and dead babies: Pregnancy and pregnancy loss in analysis," Ana Teresa Vale, through two clinical examples, provides us with a reflection on pregnancy losses and their repercussions. Pregnancy loss takes a toll not only on patients, but also on the analyst, leaving the analytic field invaded by dead babies and intoxicated by the death drive. This situation will demand a working-through of painful emotions and fantasies that, if successful, will allow growth and transformation.

Conceição Tavares de Almeida in her chapter "As good as it gets: Psychoanalysis as a fertile encounter" draws an analogy between the patient's infertility and the direness we can find on the analytic field in some situations. Through the presentation of clinical vignettes, the author addresses the pain experienced in the face of infertility, which is projected in the analyst, making the analytic field sterile, dire, monotonous. The working-through of this pain and the fantasies associated with infertility will then generate a fertile analytical encounter.

In the chapter "The taboo of egg donation: From fairy tales to myth," Sofia Barandiaran explores the taboos linked to motherhood, specifically the taboo surrounding egg donation, which often remains a well-kept secret, never shared with anyone, on the part of the couples who resort to it. The need to resort to donated eggs triggers a set of fantasies in women, intricated with their childhood history and psychic dynamics, fantasies that are explored and deepened in this chapter. Resorting to her clinical practice, the author also shows the usefulness of analysis for the elaboration of these fantasies.

The issue of egg donation continues to be addressed in the next chapter, this time from the point of view of its possible impact on the establishment of the mother-baby bond. In "Symbolic affiliation in an egg donor case," Renata Viola Vives makes a detailed description of a child psychoanalysis with a boy generated from an egg donation and the impact this had on the parental couple and on the child. Based on this clinical illustration, the author develops the problem associated with symbolic affiliation – every baby, whatever its origin, has to be symbolically adopted and integrated into a generational chain. In some cases of egg donation, this process of symbolic adoption and affiliation can become more challenging, and if that is the case, the role of the psychoanalyst will then be to facilitate this process.

For her part, Christine Anzieu-Premmereur, in "Motherhood without pregnancy: Surrogacy, a challenge for femininity and maternal preoccupation," addresses the issue of the development of primary maternal preoccupation when pregnancy does not take place in the body of the woman who will assume the place and function of a mother. Conflicts around feelings of guilt and debt are specifically addressed, which are always unconsciously present in any pregnancy but can become particularly challenging in cases of surrogacy. For the author, being able to give oneself the legitimacy to be a mother is connected with the development of primary maternal concern, so essential for the mother-baby bond and for the mother's attunement with her baby.

It is also with the theme of surrogate motherhood that we end the book. The last chapter, by Katy Bogliatto, is titled "Working with surrogate mothers and intended families," where the author describes the structure she has built in the organization of which she is a part, working simultaneously with the future surrogate and intended parental couple. This chapter addresses the role of the psychoanalyst in the evaluation process, in the preparation of the parental project, and in the follow-up of the pregnancy. The analyst then appears as a third party in this relationship between couple and surrogate, positioning herself in a transitional or potential space where elaborations can be made and where new elements can emerge.

Although some material on these topics has already been written and published in psychoanalytic journals in different languages, there are few published books that focus specifically on the subject of infertility, and the ones published tend to be from a sole author or a group of authors coming from the same country or region.

On the contrary, this book covers a wider spectrum of psychoanalytic traditions. Our authors come from different countries, with different cultural backgrounds, and having been trained in different schools of thought within the psychoanalytic field. Therefore, each author has her own approach, and as such a diversity of psychoanalytic theories and models are put to work to understand and help to elaborate the experiences, fantasies, and emotions resulting from infertility and AR procedures.

The issues raised by AR will appear more and more frequently in our offices as technology will continue to evolve, bringing new solutions (and new questions), and psychoanalytic theory will have to follow this evolution. This is the aim of this book, to explore, question, and hypothesize different ways of thinking psychoanalytically about this wide topic.

References

Alkolombre, P. (2008). *Deseo de hijo, pasión de hijo*. Letra Viva.

Alkolombre, P. (2023). *The desire and passion for a child - Psychoanalysis and contemporary reproductive techniques*. Routledge.

Ansermet, F. (2017). *The art of making children – The new world of assisted reproductive technology*. Routledge.

Deutsch, H. (1960). *A Psicologia da Mulher: Maternidade*. Losada.

Chatel, M. (1995). *Mal estar na procriação: As mulheres e a medicina da reprodução*. Editora Campo Matêmico.

Faure-Pragier, S. (2003). *Les bébés de l'inconscient - Le psychanalyste face aux stérilités féminines aujourd'hui*. Presses Universitaries de France.

Faure-Pragier, S. (2008). La sterilité feminine peut-elle être considerée comme une affection psychosomatique?, *Carnet Psy*, *127*: 39–43. Available online https://www.cairn.info/revue-le-carnet-psy-2008-5-page-39.htm

Keenan, L. (2023). OMS alerta que 1 em cada 6 pessoas é afetada pela infertilidade em todo o mundo. *Organização Pan-Americana da Saúde*, 4 de abril de 2023. Available online https://www.paho.org/pt/noticias/4-4-2023-oms-alerta-que-1-em-cada-6-pessoas-e-afetada-pela-infertilidade-em-todo-mundo

Langer, M. (1981). *Maternidade e sexo*. Editora Artes Médicas.

Leon, I. (1996). Reproductive loss: Barriers to psychoanalytic treatment. *Journal of the American Academy of Psychoanalysis*, *24*: 341–352.

Mann, M. (2014). *Psychoanalytic aspects of assisted reproductive technology*. Routledge.

Marion, P. (2022). *Sexuality and procreation in the age of biotechnology – Desire and its discontents*. Routledge.

Pines, D. (1972). Pregnancy and motherhood: Interaction between fantasy and reality. *British Journal of Medical Psychology*, *45*: 333–343. https://doi.org/10.1111/j.2044-8341.1972.tb02216.x

Queiroz, C. (2023). Em 45 anos, fertilização in vitro gera mais de dez milhões de bebés no mundo. *Folha de São Paulo*, 23 de julho de 2023. Available online in https://www1.folha.uol.com.br/equilibrioesaude/2023/07/em-45-anos-fertilizacao-in-vitro-gera-mais-de-10-milhoes-de-bebes-no-mundo.shtml

Ramirez-Galvez (2007). Corpos fragmentados e domesticados. *Cadernos Pagu 33*: 83–115.

Raphael-Leff, J. (2013). 'Opening shut doors' – The emotional impact of infertility and therapeutic issues. In E. Quagliata (Ed.) *Becoming parents, overcoming obstacles*. (pp. 83–108). Karnac.

Vives, R. (2021). *Ensaios sobre reprodução assistida, parentalidades e adoção*. Gênese.

Vives, R. (2022). *Ensaios sobre reprodução assistida, parentalidades e adoção – volume 2*. Gênese.

Chapter 2

Fantasies of origin and the origin of fantasies

Paola Marion, with contributions from Eleonora Di Lucia, Veronika Garms, Selene Mancinelli, and Giovanna Pavanello

Introduction

As is well known, resorting to technical solutions is no longer simply a matter of facing infertility and thus linked to strictly therapeutic aims. For some time, although with appreciable differences between the various geographical, cultural, and social contexts, there has also been recourse to the procreative biotechnologies to address and meet other types of request and other demands which prompt us to envisage an extension of medicine and science capable of answering and "satisfying" ever broader requirements and desires. This is testified by the constant rise in the age of women who are resorting to assisted reproductive technology (ART) and who hope, thanks to technology, that they will be able to overcome the limits imposed on our body by biology. To this are added the requests coming from lone women who, despite not having a partner, are not inclined to give up on motherhood, from homosexual couples, from transgender people.[1] The horizon is widening, giving rise to composite schemata with the entry of multiple figures who come together on the project.

These new scenarios, which go beyond the boundaries of the traditional triangle, prompt us to think about our origins, *where we start from*, a theme that extends through the life of every human individual and of which Eliot gives us a dazzling description in the closing passage of *East Coker*: "Home is where one starts from. As we grow older/ The world becomes stranger, the pattern more complicated/ Of dead and living". Winnicott (1986) replaces the Cartesian "*Cogito, ergo sum*" with "*Sum*, I am" to describe the sense of unity which every subject needs in order to set off into that "pattern more complicated" that is existence. He refers to the sense of basic unity, a sense that concerns our identity, biological and physical as much as emotional and psychological, and "the development towards independence and ever-new meanings to the concept of wholeness" (p. 56).

The caregiver's unconscious contents infiltrate the processes of attachment and nurturing of the child, as Laplanche (2007) has also taught us via the concepts of "enigmatic message" and "fundamental anthropological condition". The lived experiences of the new modes of procreation and birth, the

DOI: 10.4324/9781032693446-2

movements and unconscious fantasies that accompany these choices, if they are not integrated into a meaningful context (Marion, 2016a), can reach the child as an "extra", a mysterious and impenetrable content, a sort of "unthought known" (Bollas, 1987) that alters and complicates the sense of unity of the Self which Winnicott talks about. When this happens (although it is by no means certain that it *will* happen) it may give rise to complex psychic processes that challenge the representational capacities and emotional resources of the subjects involved.

We draw on some clinical cases to offer a reflection on the fantasies, both those of the children and their parents, which accompany the questions about origins and which we have encountered specifically in cases of heterologous fertilization of lone mothers and in one case of an insemination that took place many years after the embryos had been frozen. No clinical experience can be generalised, and our observations – as is the case in any psychoanalytic experience – refer only to what we have encountered in our clinical practice and through our attention to the underlying unconscious processes. Empirical research conducted on larger numbers and with different instruments can present results that do not coincide with our reflections (Imrie, Jadva & Golombok, 2020; Golombok, Jones, Hall, Foley, Imrie & Jadva, 2023). It must be recognized, however, that in these cases the investigation addresses fields of observation and uses other instruments, whereas the psychoanalyst's attention is directed towards understanding the troubles of those who consult us, towards the investigation of the unconscious movements and meanings underlying the symptoms and the manifest discourse.

In this universe, reminiscent of the "technological vertigo" that Ansermet (2015) writes about, the conditions of procreation change and the bond of the sexual union between a man and a woman vanishes. Along with this, there is also a diminution of the profound, one-to-one mind-body relationship which – as we will see – is reflected in the way we work out our origins. Indeed, the very term psychosexuality, introduced by psychoanalysis, refers to the rooting of the psyche in the body and how there are deep processes in human sexuality and in its various manifestations associated with corporeality, relatedness, the instinctual drive, desire, and affectivity. And all these levels contribute to the subjective constitution of an identity and to the identificatory processes.

The unconscious alliances which found the familial nucleus, the couple, and the family and define the relation between generations are infused with the organisation of sexuality (Kaës, 2009). The disjunction between procreative practices and sexuality, the entry onto the scene of protagonists other than the two partners, the medicalisation of a process considered natural and intimate, and the interplay of more and more complicated variables raise questions about the outcomes and effects on the fantasy level. And it raises questions about how this affects the fantasies and the imaginative elaboration of all those involved, especially the most vulnerable subjects, the children. It is on these topics that this chapter concentrates.

The place of origin

The topic of the search for one's origin characterizes a foundational myth of psychoanalysis, that of Oedipus. "However base my birth, I must know about it" (Sophocles, 2002, *Oedipus Rex*, ver. 157, p. 33), he states in the tragedy, thus revealing the powerful drive within each one of us to shed light on our beginnings. We know how the Oedipus myth, like a musical theme, has been reprised and reinvented many times through the history of psychoanalysis. From being a sexual model it has undergone a gradual transformation to become a model of knowledge, as Bion (1967) has taught us. In this interpretation the "sexual crime" becomes a peripheral element. The accent shifts onto the impulse to know (K) and the conflicts that this generates. In this sense we may say that Oedipus is a myth of knowledge and searching that tells us about the attempt to know and the attempt to deny a knowledge that is too traumatic (Abadi, 1978; Marion, 1991). The journey of Oedipus speaks to us about the journey in search of his own identity, the role of the fantasies in play which involve all the actors in the field and extend back to the generations who came before us.

Winnicott (1965) writes that "it is not possible to understand the attitude of parents to their children apart from the consideration of the meaning of each child in terms of the parents' conscious and unconscious fantasy around the act that produced the conception" (p. 61). The child's conscious and unconscious fantasies related to the primal scene and also the parents' conscious and unconscious fantasies, not only about that child before and after conception, but also about having decided to resort to assisted reproduction, influence each other and constitute the background and nucleus which makes possible the dream of one's own life-project and one's own sexuality. The place of origin, *where we start from* in his words, is thus located in the desire and the fantasies which accompany the mind of the potential parents when they think about making a baby and which constitute the dream which everyone has about their child.

The emotional and imaginative working-through which accompanies the journey of bringing a new creature to life involves sexuality first of all, reactivates the oedipal and pre-oedipal dilemmas, arousing in the second phase, that of adult sexuality, quanta of unconscious fantasies and conflicts linked to infantile sexuality. This earlier sexuality is a dimension which infuses psychic life throughout our existence, functions as the source of desire and as a creative impulse, and can be triggered into awakening itself in crucial episodes. Besides, infantile sexuality represents the place of origin of life's central questions and the desire to know and explore, as first Freud taught us in Little Hans ([1909] 1977), and Klein after him. The riddle of riddles – "where do babies come from?"; "where do I come from?" – accompanies infantile curiosity, and the answers that the child comes up with to these basic questions constitute the "theories about birth" or "infantile sexual theories" which, as we well know, can take a variety of different forms (Marion, 2016a, 2017). These are questions and theories traditionally attached to the parental couple and their sexuality.

For psychoanalysis, the *primal scene*, before and outside us, represents the starting point of the oedipal scenario around which the fantasies of origin are structured. The parents' sexuality constitutes the mystery, the secret place, with which the child is confronted and which gives rise to powerful feelings and emotions of curiosity, exclusion, envy, rivalry. Today it is perhaps not as mysterious and secret as it once was, the present world being one in which children are surrounded by a hypertrophic production of images (Riolo, 2005) about bodies and the various manifestations of sexuality.

However, the unconscious translation of all this is never direct, and while we can agree with Ansermet (2015) that in the unconscious the couple is still the father and mother rather than the sexual man-woman couple, there is a point of origin which is central in influencing the quality of subsequent fantasies and our elaboration of them and of our own history. I am referring to the element of pleasure, to its greater or lesser presence, which we connect, if not ideally then at least as far as possible, to the sexual scene that acts as the background of our roots (Marion, 2016b). Sexual desire, as distinct from the category of needs, is characterized by "ecstasy in mutual enjoyment" (Green, 1995, p. 877). This is a pleasure that has its roots in the body and in bodies in relation to each other and is reflected in desire for the other. The pleasure experienced in the area of sexuality and in the couple-relation will be extended to and colour the pleasure felt towards the child, permeating conception, if it happens, and after the nurture and care.

Indeed, the adult and the parental couple are not confined to satisfying the infant's needs, but act as a source of pleasure, bodily in the first instance, which becomes a foundational experience of the child's being, sense of self, and vital project. As Seulin (2015) writes, "autoerotic infantile sexuality therefore appears as a second phase of the sexual in the infant, whereas the first phase of sexuality unfolds in the presence of the object and via an affective sharing with it" (pp. 56–57). Seulin's assertion clearly underlines the importance of the couple's desire, for each other and for the child, their world of fantasy which accompanies the child's conception and growth. So, if our roots go down into this desire that precedes us (the desire of the couple), into a primal scene and into a time that precedes us, the beginning will cast its shadow or its light onto the fantasies we will have about our origins, about our idea of ourselves and the relation between us and our body.

The new forms of procreation challenge the modes of birth traditionally located in the parental couple, "overturning all differences, both sexual and temporal" (Ansermet, 2015, p. 54), and above all expel the sexual union from the act of conception, replacing it with concrete procedures and a predominance of the real over the psychic. We can have children with people of the same sex, with unknown donors, and by using cryopreserved embryos or the uterus of another woman. The doctors who aid procreation can be invested with sexual fantasies and become fantasy-figures in a "medically assisted adultery" (*ibid.*, p. 83); in fantasy, the figures of the donors can be helpers or invested with the potency that the partner lacks, and so on. Each of these situations presents a variety of scenarios which define the place of origin in an equally diverse way, one that prompts psychoanalytic thinking.

The questions raised by heterological fertilization – who is the other? – are extended into the questions and fantasies about one's own origin: "who am I?"; "where do I come from?" The answer can be even more traumatic than the question because donors (where it is possible to know them) are not included in the parental set-up and do not acknowledge themselves as biological mothers and fathers. Where surrogate pregnancy is necessary, it further complicates the panorama and adds a new aspect. In this regard, ART goes far beyond the goals of treatment and extend into uncharted territory. It is a matter of incorporating the presence of other figures who only have life on the fantasy level but have contributed to conception in various roles and functions: genetic parts of unknown donors, women who have undertaken pregnancy for others, the doctor or medical team in itself, and even a combination of such processes. Or else, as we were saying earlier, there is a need to deal with times before fertilization and the start of pregnancy, as with cryopreserved embryos waiting for the right moment to be implanted.

As Ehrenhaft (2014) postulates, the triangle is enlarged, becomes a square, a pentagon, even a hexagon, within an ever-expanding circle. We are entering the sphere of stories linked to mythology and religions, rich in accounts of the most bizarre ways of coming into the world (Ansermet, 2019), or the sphere of infantile sexual theories which construct fantasy scenarios, in the often anxious search for an answer to the riddle of their origin.

Parsons (2014) says that working through the idea of our beginning – just like that of our end – has a profound significance for every one of us and requires "a lifelong psychic work" (p. 21). And the work that the protagonists of these experiences are called upon to do really is hard. The types of fantasy linked to these places of origin, which thus become fantasies about origin, are described in the cases to which we will refer, involving children born by recourse to heterologous fertilization on the part of lone mothers.

The origin of fantasies

In the case of Stella,[2] a seven-year-old girl, the story of her conception takes the therapist into a climate of incredulity and dismay. At the age of 45, Stella's mother Carmela decides to give herself a "present". She travels to a foreign country to freeze her ova without her current partner's knowledge. Seven of them are produced. The ova are fertilized with the semen which her partner nevertheless is willing to provide, and the embryos are subsequently frozen. Many family vicissitudes take up Carmela's attention and mental space. Time passes and it is only at the age of 54, fully nine years later, that Carmela travels abroad again to the clinic storing the embryos and has them implanted.

They thaw three of the original seven and, after a careful examination, decide to implant the most "vital", Stella. Despite the woman's age the implanting goes well. In the meantime, her partner has gone. At 31 weeks a serious complication is diagnosed in the pregnancy and an emergency caesarean section is carried out to save both mother and child. Stella is born and placed in intensive care. She is brought up by her mother and referred for therapy because she is exhibiting strange behaviour at school: she massages her friend's private parts, masturbates herself, or asks her friends to let her pee on their hands.

In the sessions, Stella protects herself from contact with the therapist by adopting an absolutely despotic and dictatorial manner. A recurring theme in her play involves the doctor, who alternately becomes the mother, charged with the task of operating on a baby boy who cannot pee. The only possible cure is to cut off his willy. Sometimes the baby is stamped on, thrown into the various corners of the room and killed, all of which is accompanied by sadistic and disturbing laughter. The game continues and Stella brings two new children into the scene, a boy and a girl, as well as the figure of the (male) doctor who gives the children an injection of pee with germs in it and adds, "No, make 3 pricks instead of 7". The children faint and blood comes out of the girl's "front bottom". Pee recurs in the games and seems to carry connotations of seminal fluid: however, it contains germs and, although it is supposed to fertilize a body attacked with injections, it fails so badly that the body bleeds and aborts.

At a meeting, the mother tells the therapist that for her it's as if Stella is nine years older "and this is why she seems bigger than her age, it's as if she's sixteen, a bit of an adolescent already", by which the mother intends to make sense of her daughter's sexualised behaviour which takes physical form in her fantasies and games, which are all centred on the body, both male and female, on the anatomy and its functioning. Stella's very disturbing fantasies seem to reflect those of her mother about the ova frozen so many years before, which make her perceive her daughter as being conceived and "created" in a period prior to her actual gestation.

Later, she will tell the therapist how the girl is asking to meet her real mother who she is convinced exists somewhere. The mother comments that this fantasy may be because of her age, perhaps a result of "jokes" made by her classmates about having an "old" mother, as if a mother aged 61 could only be an adoptive mother, not a conceiving one. Stella's confusion, which impels her to imagine a real mother located somewhere else and an affective relationship with a different parent from the one who is present, sends its roots down into the omnipotent maternal fantasies which deny the limit and "cut out" the third represented by the paternal figure, as we also see in the girl's games. In this highly dramatic case, "assisted fertilization" seems to have inverted its function. Instead of being an opportunity to help overcome the distress and difficulty in conceiving, it is used to support an omnipotent dream which cannot take the needs and desires of the other into account, engendering profound confusion and fragmentation in the child. Thinking of what Bollas (1987) writes, we could say that "the shadow of the object" and its choices has fallen on Stella.

This highly dramatic case touches on a very delicate point. The place of origin can be interfered with and violently compromised by omnipotent fantasies, which often hide an auto-generative fantasy and gain the upper hand over the examination of reality. Winnicott (1988) writes that the primal scene is "the basis of individual stability" (p. 64) because it enables the child to realise the dream of taking the place of one of the two partners and makes possible "the sorting out of what is called reality and fantasy" (ibid.). The flesh-and-blood child, who resorts to a complex symptomatology in order to express her troubled state, represents the reminder of reality which asserts itself against the denial of time which the woman seems to be making through her decisions.

Something similar happens to Vittorio, a four-year-old boy conceived by heterological fertilization and brought up by a lone mother, without a flesh-and-blood father. It is the mother, Laura,[3] who asks for psychotherapeutic help at the same time as Vittorio starts kindergarten. The beginning of this experience of school is difficult for both of them, a decisive moment of separation. Vittorio was born via heterologous fertilization which took place in another country. Laura was a lone woman and at that time had just ended a romantic relationship with a man with whom she had thought she would be able to have children. In retracing the fertilization journey, she talks about how easy, possible, and quick it all seemed to her. This feeling was increased by the success of the first implantation attempt. She wonders in *après-coup* if it might have been necessary at that delicate moment to talk to a psychologist because nobody prepared her properly for what came after: the contact with a real baby and all the struggles that one goes through with a small child.

Vittorio asks his mother where his father is and Laura, for her part, feels she does not have the internal equipment for answering this question. Moreover, in Laura's history there is a father who abandons his family and a mother who brings up her daughters on her own. Laura had resorted to ART with a desire for a pregnancy of her own, and for a motherhood that might be able to inject vitality and a future into a difficult and painful life story. She had also nursed the illusion that Vittorio would be exclusively grateful to his mother for having given him life, while the boy, probably observing his peers with different family set-ups, was starting to draw his mother onto slippery terrain for her.

In the sessions, Laura finds it hard to imagine that her son will be capable of desiring a father not only as an abstract entity, but also as a bodily presence: a father who plays, who says no, who is loving, and lays down rules. Faced with her son's insistence that he wants to know who caused him to be born, Laura lets herself be guided by a book on the subject: there is a place where lots of generous men give their semen and Mummy took some and he was born. Vittorio gets agitated, asks his mother to close the book, becomes rejecting. Amongst the book's illustrations, there is a woman almost casually pointing to a container of semen, and then the same woman is shown waiting for a baby to be born. The image in the book, representing a woman alone with no one at her side, choosing the seed that will fertilize her, seems to exalt an idea of female omnipotence that frightens the child.

Vittorio seems opposed to the thought that this is his place of origin, the thought of a mother who is so big and powerful. The boy seems to be high-lighting an absence in the chain of generations into which he has been inserted, missing a parental couple as a space in which desire is cultivated. He will say, "hasn't Daddy got onto a ship? And now maybe he can't get off again".

As the work with Laura proceeds, the therapist discovers the intensity of Vittorio's search. The mother's choice of conception has deleted the other's corporeality while Vittorio, albeit in his imagination, gives a father's body back to his mother. For example, hearing a male voice telling children a story, Vittorio comments that this is how he imagines a father's voice. Then he asks his mother to act out a story and perform several of the characters. Seeing how hard and tiring it is for her to move from one role to the next, he exclaims, "We really need a Daddy".

The complexity of these places of origin originates equally complex fanta-sies, and all the characters in the scene are involved in a network of feelings about an absence, that of the donor whom they would like to deny, but whose ghost repeatedly returns, like Banquo, especially via the children. The intricate fabric of relations offered by these situations with their marked genetic asym-metry and the anxiety that accompanies them, often make it almost impossible to think about them. As Ehrenhaft (2014) writes, "when any of those inner shapes are destroyed, denied, or compromised, the child is at risk of being left with a void in relatedness or an anxiety about the bonds to one or both intended parents" (p. 30).

As Laura says to her therapist, it is the parents themselves, if they have no one alongside them, who underestimate the emotional charge entailed in bring-ing an unknown person into the intimacy of conception and ought to know about how that unknown person will leave his or her own "genetic imprint" on the child who is to be born. The parents' unmetabolized fantasies about their choices are transmitted to the children, who may find themselves facing an unfillable void, like Vittorio, or an unrepresented figure translated into dra-matic symptoms, as in Stella.

The difficulty in working through this process and the dissociation that may be created in the parents' minds can be traced in situations where the parents choose to keep origins secret, not only from their own son or daughter but also from the extended family. Recourse to ART seems to generate feelings of shame and guilt about one's sexual and procreative inadequacy or about choices that may reveal fantasies of infantile omnipotence. The silence indi-cates the defence of a private nucleus that cannot be made accessible to others, but neither can it be worked through within the parents themselves. The prob-lems which the parent or parents may have with mentally and emotionally inte-grating the process they have gone through is reflected in the child, who no longer, and not only, has to deal with two parents who leave him or her outside the bedroom, but with presences which have never entered the bedroom. The place of origin is fraught with troubling phantoms and, for the children who feel that they are the depository of a secret about how they were conceived or the revelation of a partial truth which conceals a piece of the story – the unspoken that prompts Oedipus to make his journey to Delphi – acts as a crack that can threaten and undermine the sense of their own personal experience, their psychic and emotional growth.

The fantasies of origin

An example of what Bogliatto and De Vriet-Goldmann (2019) call "clinical practice in extreme cases" ("*clinique de l'extrême*") or "clinical practice in the abyss" ("*clinique de l'abîme*"), in which infantile omnipotence predominates and it is impossible to mourn the fantasies of immortality, seems to be represented by the case of Nadia and Rafael,[4] who confront the therapist with a situation right at the extreme; so extreme as to seriously compromise Rafael's growth, and above all the development of his symbolic capacities.

A foreign woman comes to the therapist's consulting room, a lone mother over 50 who will be in Italy for a short time and is seeking help for her three-year-old son. She describes him as simultaneously tyrannical, incomprehensible, and unreachable. He is not yet talking, goes to sleep late in the evening and always in her bed, is adamant in his refusals, eats when and where he wants. Nadia's language is concrete and seems not to express emotions; a very strong sense of foreignness and loneliness predominates. The feeling she communicates to the therapist is that Rafael has been brought to her (therapist) like a "broken" object which can only be repaired by the hands of an expert.

The boy was born via a double donation of gametes (sperm and ova) in a distant country. Nadia went through pregnancy on her own, in solitude, and couldn't imagine her child in any way; in her thoughts she only begged him to not pass through her vagina but be born by caesarean, which is what actually happened. Faced with this account, the therapist feels catapulted into an *elsewhere* where there is nothing familiar to cling to: there is an incomprehensible child conceived in a foreign country from alien gametes, and even the language used by the doctor and Nadia is foreign, third, a language which is not the mother tongue for either of them. The therapist decides that undertaking treatment for the child alone is not the right solution. Leaving the mother out would confirm her fear of being unable to "generate" something good and would confirm her conviction that, in matters concerning her generativity, she must always delegate to others more powerful than her, such as the donors who have enabled her to conceive.

A joint mother–child therapy is offered, alternating with individual meetings with Nadia to reflect together on what happens in the exchanges with the child. This is a way to acknowledge the need for psychic and emotional "nesting", which the procedures of assisted heterologous fertilization together with Nadia's personal circumstances had prevented, and to which the chosen mode of therapy might be an answer. The therapy may offer this mother a time/place for repairing the psychic skin that envelops mother-child, thereby activating her inner resources, a time/place to bring about the psychic and bodily work that had been missing in the time and place of conception and pregnancy.

The absence of an imaginary child during pregnancy or the difficulty in imagining him/her, which we have found in our experiences with heterologous fertilization, takes the form of a psychic paralysis, which can offer protection from feelings of death and loss related to the experience of infertility and often also to abortions, while, on the other hand, showing how the possibility of believing in one's own generative capacities has been violently compromised. The lack of fantasies about the baby which have been replaced by a sort of freezing or by experiences of anxiety, is ascribable to the absence of a known, familiar place of origin where one can dwell and give birth to a continuity between body and psyche, between psychic and physical pregnancy, a place for generating *rêveries*. In this respect we agree with what Bogliatto and De Vriet-Goldmann (2019) state regarding to the need to "think the unthinkable" (p. 4). In heterologous fertilization, indeed, patients are confronted with the challenging task of trying to think about the void of origins, and their defensive reactions seem to allow them to survive in this "waste land" (T. S. Eliot), waiting for better times.

The therapeutic work with Nadia and Rafael was fortunately very fruitful. The boy began to interact with his environment, played games in which there was space for the other and accompanied them with his first words. Mother and child found each other in their own way and enjoyed it. In Nadia's individual sessions, mother and therapist repeatedly went through Rafael's story, his conception and birth, the first months, and the paralysing fears that Nadia had experienced in those early moments. One day, on her PC she shows her therapist the donors' profiles, Rafael's biological mother and father, explaining her reasons for choosing them. It is a moving moment for them both, evidence of the fabric they have woven and the start of a story that can now begin to be told.

This clinical example witnesses the importance of listening to and thinking about what these patients put inside of us in the form of projections, about their painful and persecutory experiences for which we become the depositories. These are experiences linked not only to the battle to overcome the sense of death caused by the failure of their generative capacities and the narcissistic wound of infertility, but also to the intrusive and persecutory nature of the procedures, and especially the idea of hosting such presences (donors, surrogate mothers, gynaecologists, medical doctors of various kinds), that may be felt as alien and unknown in the most profound, sexual, and psychic intimacy.

As a consequence of these painful and intrusive experiences, these patients' speech can appear and sound concrete and rigid, accompanied by a paralysis of thought and fantasy activity. As Bogliatto and De Vriet-Goldmann (2019, p. 11) write, the lacuna in these patients' work of symbolisation would thus be experienced first in the 'body-to-body' encounter between the patient and the analyst, who becomes the place for expelling the excess of quantitative charge and the lack of qualitative translation, associated with the act of ART.

Here it is as if the children, babies or younger ones, as well as adolescents, take over the task of drawing others' attention to the disease, developing symptoms or fantasies which grasp the problematic nature of the place of their origin.

This is what happens, for example, with Elizabeth, a seven-year-old girl, the only child of a lone mother, conceived abroad by heterologous FIVET (fertilization in vitro and embryo transfer).[5] They came to the doctor with a recommendation for psychotherapy following an assessment carried out in a hospital clinic, which identified that the girl was inhibited in play and in the use of fantasy and imaginative thought. From a very early age, Elizabeth has displayed furious tantrums which cause her mother more and more distress, until she asks to be killed or states that she intends to kill herself. Elizabeth suffers because she feels alone and isolated, despite the rich and varied social context created around her: she observes children playing while she seems to be shut out.

At the first meeting, as soon as Elizabeth enters the therapy room, she sits at the table and creates her own identity card, writes her first name and surname on it, draws herself with a tail and draws a small animal alongside the self-portrait, telling the therapist that animals are her family. The therapist is surprised by Elizabeth's ability to hand over her problem, to lead her to the essence of the enigmatic cruxes needing to be untied, and the fantasies about her origin and identity. Elizabeth's mother has not yet found the words to share her daughter's story with her, and the child has never allowed herself to pose questions about her origin in such a way as to give form to the figure of an absent father. The encounter seems to reveal the girl's desire to pass through a closed door inside herself and to discover what is behind her feelings of emptiness, difference, and foreignness, behind the furious reactions which have brought her to this consultation: "who am I?"; "where do I come from?"

Elizabeth doesn't feel she is a child amongst children: as she says herself, she feels that animals are her family. The girl's fantasies about her family romance are introduced by the story of the princess and the dragon that she tells in the session: although she is happy with everything she has, on her birthday the princess asks not to feel alone anymore. She is given a little dragon to keep her company and – after various vicissitudes and adventures – it leads the princess to her real home, where a mother and a father happily welcome her. The question/request which Elizabeth puts to her therapist/dragon by means of the fairy tale seems to be asking for a companion on a journey that may set free her fantasies and transform her feelings, so that she can begin to build an inner couple, a representation of the parental couple, at her origin. The theme of identity and origins acts as a compass orienting the journey, which unfolds in a variety of ways.

One topic which soon emerges is time. Elizabeth makes it clear that she is disturbed by the ticking of the clock in the therapy room, which the analyst initially associates with the time of the *setting*, defining and limiting the pleasure of being together. She gradually forms the impression that the patient wants to communicate something else. The girl tells her about a squirrel that she came across in a park during a walk with her mother. They couldn't stop to watch it because "we were in a hurry. It was such a pity!" The girl's life is highly animated, marked out by often frenetic activities; there is always something to do. The therapist associates this temporal rhythm with those that are marked out by a metronome, and she comments on the girl's desire to linger over experiences, her wish for a temporal dimension accompanied by the pleasure of a time enjoyed together. As a result of this interpretation, Elizabeth introduces the game of a lioness stretched out suckling her young, a game characterized by the silence and the sensation of contact that is created. The "magical" moment is abruptly interrupted by the game of the roundabout. Elizabeth comments that the roundabout "goes round death" and on the top of it there is a girl who falls but lives. Then she goes back to the game with the lioness who scolds her cubs for being greedy and tells them to be careful with what they eat: "there may be dangerous DNA that's bad for you".

Reflecting on Elizabeth's fantasy of suspending the flow of time and experiencing intimate moments of calm, but also reflecting on the deadly fantasies linked to the dangerous DNA, the therapist realises how the girl's origin lacked a time of pleasure experienced within the couple. Instead, there was a conception dogged by the rushing of the biological clock and rhythms marked out by medical protocols, a conception accompanied by deadly feelings linked to the presence of something uncontrollable and dangerous inside her (DNA). Elizabeth's fantasy of finding a time that is intensely enjoyed with her therapist, in a pleasant emotional atmosphere, may refer to the desire to write a new primal scene.

Conclusions

In our opinion, the questions and fantasies at the heart of these experiences are well described by the brief clinical cases we have presented. If the primal scene changes, what kind of fantasy is activated? In what way is this reflected in the questions about origin that we all ask ourselves and engrave into our biographical story?

The changes introduced by biotechnologies touch the deep nucleus of our identity and modify the primary, founding relational schemata. In these situations the desire for a child is no longer a desire that needs and encounters the other's desire in order to bring a third to life, but a desire which sometimes appears so determined to fulfil its wish that it reveals itself as an infantile fantasy of omnipotence.

Over its long years of life, psychoanalysis has shown us how the intrapsychic is born and develops in the light of the interpsychic – both are intrinsically interwoven (Bolognini, 2019). The psychic space of subjects involved in ART is inhabited by a multitude of places and figures, and this affects the weaving of fantasies that takes place between parents and children. A *fil rouge* seems to link all these experiences, from the slightest to the most extreme, which is the shifting of one's personal centre of gravity to *an elsewhere* (Marion, 2017). The *elsewhere* is the tear in the foundation of origin that may be left open, as much in the child as in the parents, and may turn into a family secret.

Nevertheless, as the clinical accounts show, the force of the infantile sexuality that represents the dimension of curiosity and desire is not silenced and seems to go on weaving its thread, looking for a place and time to express itself. In fantasy and play, or by producing symptoms, children express the search for that *elsewhere*, show their attempts to give it shape and representation, to find answers, and address an "unsaid" which confronts them with something about themselves and their roots that is hard to think about, something that will influence the construction of their family romance. Therapeutic work and the encounter with the analyst constitute the place and time where an alien *elsewhere* can start to be transformed into a habitable space and open new channels of personal and creative investment.

The setting and the psychoanalytic listening meet both the parents' need to finally feel their child as their own, as the cases of Laura or Nadia show, and the children's need, as for Vittorio and Elizabeth, for the silence on their origins to be gradually lifted. Not only this: it is also a space where, in the presence of a listening other, patients try to recover those bodily and sensory dimensions that were missing (see Laura and Vittorio), replaced by artificial procedures, or try to recover a time (see Elizabeth or Rafael) when there was pleasure in the encounter rather than the *timing* of medical protocols. It can therefore provide "a safe autonomous place for the ongoing discovery and repair of the self" (Apfel and Keylor, 2002, p. 98–99). Giving meaning to our beginning is not only a "lifelong psychic work" as Parsons says, and a very hard work, but also the premise for everyone to create one's own history and write one's own future.

Notes

1 Recourse to gamete donation, the freezing of ova while the woman is still fertile in the expectation of using them in some unspecified future, the freezing of embryos for subsequent transfer, to which is added surrogate motherhood, open up scenarios that no longer, and not only, concern the desire to resist the destiny of infertility which is held to be unjustly punitive – as it was for women in the Bible – but prompt ideas about an extreme extension of the ability of medicine and science to achieve any ambition.
2 The case was treated by Dr. Selene Mancinelli.
3 The case was treated by Dr. Eleonora Di Lucia.
4 The case was treated by Dr. Veronika Garms.
5 The case was treated by Dr. Giovanna Pavanello.

References

Abadi, M. (1978). Meditazione su (l') Edipo. *Rivista di Psicoanalisi*, 24: 391–424.

Ansermet, F. (2015). *La fabrication des enfants. Un vertige technologique*. Odile Jacob. (English Translation, *The Art of Making Children: The new world of Assisted Reproductive Technology*, Routledge, 2018).

Ansermet F. (2019). *L'origine à venir*. Diderot.

Apfel, R. & Keylor, R. (2002). Psychoanalysis and infertility. Myths and realities. *International Journal of Psychoanalysis*, 83: 85–104. DOI: https://doi.org/10.1516/4089-JBCW-YNT8-QTCM

Bion, W. (1967). *Second thoughts*. William Heinemann Medical Books.

Bogliatto, K. & De Vriet-Goldmann, C. (2019). Parentalités. Origines et procréation médicalement assistée. Aspects psychanalytiques. *International Journal of Psychoanalysis Open*, 6, 20: 1–31. Available online https://www.psynem.org/Perinatalite/Personnes_pratiques_lieux/PMA

Bollas C. (1987). *The Shadow of the Object. Psychoanalysis of the Unthought Known*. Free Association Books.

Bolognini, S. (2019). Vital flows between the self and non-self. The interpsychic. Routledge, 2022.

Ehrensaft, D. (2014). Family complexes and oedipal circles: Mothers, fathers, babies, donors and surrogates. In M. Mann (Ed.). *Psychoanalytic aspects of Assisted Reproductive Technology* (pp. 19–43). Routledge.

Freud, S. ([1909] 1977). Analysis of a phobia of a five year old boy. In *The Pelican Freud Library, Volume 8* (pp. 169–306). Pelican Books.

Golombok, S., Jones, C., Hall, P., Foley, S., Imrie, S., & Jadva, V. (2023). A longitudinal study of families formed through third-party assisted reproduction: Mother-child relationships and child adjustment from infancy to adulthood. *Developmental psychology*, 59 (6): 1059–1073. https://doi.org/10.1037/dev0001526

Green, A. (1995). Has sexuality anything to do with psychoanalysis? *International Journal of Psychoanalysis*, 76: 871–883.

Imrie, S., Jadva, V., & Golombok, S. (2020). "Making the child mine": Mothers' thoughts and feelings about the mother-infant relationship in egg donation families. *Journal of family psychology: Journal of the Division of Family Psychology of the American Psychological Association*, 34 (4): 469–479. https://doi.org/10.1037/fam0000619

Kaës, R. (2009). *Les alliances inconscientes*. Dunod.

Laplanche, J. (2007). *Sexuel. La sexualité élargie au sens freudien 2000–2006*. Presses Universitaires de France.

Marion (1991). L'Edipo Re tra mito e tragedia. In C. Bollas (Ed.) *Perché Edipo? Intorno mito e alla tragedia*. (pp. 47–61). Borla.

Marion, P. (2016a). Infantile sexuality and Freud's legacy. *International Journal of Psychoanalysis*, 97: 641–664.

Marion, P. (2016b). La logica del piacere all'origine dello psichico. *Rivista di Psicoanalisi*, 62: 845–860.

Marion, P. (2017). *Il disagio del desiderio. Sessualità e procreazione nel tempo delle biotecnologie*. Donzelli. Roma. (English Translation, *Sexuality and Procreation in the Age of Biotechnology. Desire and its discontents*, Routledge, London, New York, 2021).

Parsons, M. (2014). *Living Psychoanalysis: From Theory to Experience*. Routledge.

Riolo, F. (2005). Eidolopoiesi. *Psiche*, 2: 147–150.

Seulin, C. (2015). Émergence et transformations de la sexualité infantile dans la cure. Presented at the 75ème congrès des psychanalystes de langue française: *Le sexuel infantile et ses destins*, which was held in Lyon, 14–17 May 2015.

Sophocles (2002). *Oedipus Rex*. Perfection Learning.

Winnicott, D. (1965). *The Maturational Process and the Facilitating Environment: Studies in the Theory of Emotional Development*. Hogarth Press.

Winnicott, D. (1986). *Home is Where we Start From*. Penguin Books.

Winnicott, D. (1988). *Human Nature*. The Winnicott Trust.

Chapter 3

Illusion, illusional belief, and mourning in infertility

Emanuela Quagliata

Introduction

The emotional experience of a woman's miscarriages and her consequent fear of infertility has a significant impact on the new pregnancy and on the relationship with the new baby. A miscarriage is an invisible loss that often goes unnoticed by the people close to the patient as well as the practitioners, but it has an enormous impact that undermines the woman's sense of identity (Quagliata, 2010). It can be a traumatic event and as such represent a massive failure of the maternal capacity to contain (Garland, 1988). Miscarriages and infertility can become a confirmation of pre-existing unconscious phantasies regarding an internal object that does not give the woman permission to become a mother or can represent the most terrible betrayal on the part of the maternal object, which was supposed to protect from danger and ensure healthy development. Unresolved conflicts with the maternal internal object make the transition between being the child of one's own mother and the mother of one's own child difficult.

In this chapter I want to explore the emotional experience of some patients with infertility problems for whom the desire for motherhood had the special significance of bringing to life lost aspects of their baby-self; the non-conception consequently represented the painful failure of this vital project.

A common aspect in my patients seemed to be the fact that they had been deprived of an experience of introjection of and identification with a maternal object capable of generating and sustaining life, a 'generative mother'. The patients had been referred to me by the gynecologist who followed them to become pregnant again through assisted fertilization. After a long period of trying to procreate naturally, followed by a second phase in which they had experienced the trauma of an infertility diagnosis, they had subsequently embarked on assisted fertilization with egg donation, fulfilling their desire for motherhood with the birth of a child. However, their desire to give birth had not yet been fulfilled.

According to Raphael-Leff (2007), *generative identity* is a psychic construction of oneself as a potential progenitor. It is when the child shifts from feeling

DOI: 10.4324/9781032693446-3

like someone's creature to becoming a potential procreator in his/her own right. It takes shape during childhood, when the child recognizes and negotiates reproductive limitations such as those related to sex, generations, and the irreversibility of time. Acquisition of *generative identity* entails acknowledging and accepting one's own limitations. A shift may occur from emphasis on physical procreativity of a baby to an abstract notion of *creativity* in general.

Recognizing that parenting skills are distinct from reproductive ones allows a person to see oneself as a loving parent even with a child who is not one's own. Raphael-Leff argues that when the sense of *generative identity* remains embedded in physical reproduction, having a child becomes the central purpose of self-expression. In this case, in my opinion, the failure of reproductive capacity comes to represent the failure of one's own creativity and of the inability to make up for the lack of the introjection of a 'generative mother'.

In order to clarify what I mean by 'generative mother' I will initially refer to Bion's concept of container-contained (♀ ♂) and then place it in a broader framework concerning what in this perspective I consider a 'maternal function'.

Expanding on Klein's concept of projective identification, Bion ([1959] 1967) introduces the notion of container-contained to describe the emotional encounter between mother and baby. Bion argues that from the infant's point of view the mother should have taken into her (container), and thus experienced, the child's fear (contained) that he was dying. "It was this fear that the child could not contain [....] An understanding mother is able to experience that feeling of dread, that this baby was striving to deal with by projective identification, and yet retain a balanced outlook" (1959, p. 104). Bringing this experience back into the patient-analyst relationship, Bion argues that certain patients had to deal with a mother who could not tolerate experiencing such feelings and reacted either by denying them ingress, or alternatively by becoming prey to the anxiety which resulted from introjection of the infant's feelings.

This capacity to accommodate, understand and give meaning to primitive emotional states is attributed by Bion to the maternal *rêverie* that he considers a state of mind capable of "reception of the infant's projective identifications whether they are felt by the infant to be good or bad". (1962, p. 36). He also clarifies that the relationship between mother and child "is not with the anatomical structures only but with the *function*, not with anatomy but with physiology, not with the breast but with feeding, poisoning, loving, hating [...] with the function of providing that link between two objects" (1959, p. 102). The link Bion describes has its representation in the creative bond between parents, but also in the link between the analyst and his psychoanalytic theory in order to create thoughts, as well as in the relationship between patient and analyst which generates transformations, and in the creative relationship between the patient and his/her own thoughts.

Klein described the baby's state of mind as "a melancholia in *statu nascendi*", the time in which the baby "has to mourn the mother's breast and all that the breast and milk have come to stand for in the infant's mind: namely, love, goodness and security" ([1940] 1998, p. 345). This state of mind, known as depressive position, arises out of the Oedipal situation.

Klein (1940) expands from Freud's thinking suggesting that mourning, at any stage in life, involves re-experiencing the infantile depressive position, including loss of internal good objects of childhood, followed by the painful work of renewing and reinstating them. The losses experienced in the depressive position are not only concrete ones, such as that of the breast in weaning, but also loss of omnipotence and of an exclusive relationship to the ideal breast or mother. From this new perspective, Klein shows how the process of mourning becomes necessary and productive in development:

> Thus while grief is experienced to the full and despair is at its height, the love for the object wells up and the mourner feels more strongly that life inside and outside will go on after all and that the lost loved object can be preserved within [...] It seems that every advance in the process of mourning results in a deepening in the individual's relation to his inner objects.
>
> ([1940] 1998, p. 360)

The maternal function, therefore, involves the capacity for containment considered not a consistently available and loving mother, but as a function which also includes the presence, in the mother's mind, of the paternal qualities of setting limits, preventing an engulfing, fusional relationship; it involves her *rêverie*, which allows her to take in and give meaning to her child's feelings; as well as the presence of an oedipal triangulation in the mother's mind. This function entails her to receive and understand feelings and emotions while at the same time helping the child to process disappointments, frustrations and losses,[1] thus generating a new, deeper relationship with the child's internal and external objects. From this perspective, in my view, the introjection of an internal 'generative mother' allows the development of an identity not necessarily related to reproductive functions, but to a maternal function capable of creativity – a regenerating function after a loss.

Some authors have described how the child who is born after a perinatal loss can be regarded as a 'replacement baby' of a dead child (Reid, 2003). Therapeutic support is very helpful in mourning the loss of a child following a miscarriage and to understand the unconscious phantasy of wanting to procreate in an attempt to change the history of failed primary relationship by reversing it (Quagliata, 2010).

But we still need to further investigate what place this mourning takes in the imagination of children and parents, and if the phantasy of dead embryos interferes with the connection with the living ones. What difficulties might be encountered by parents in building the relationship with children born after an experience of infertility, and how will the child deal with scenarios concerning his/her origins? According to Joan Raphael-Leff: "the child of enigmatic self-origin may feel lost, consumed by a constant need to see without knowing what"; and "the child born out of donation, like many adopted babies, is always inserted into a place of absence, occupying a position of replacement for that which cannot be" (2003, p. 69).

I wonder about the burden that the child involved in the mother's illusion is unknowingly called to bear: to sustain the guilt of feeling necessarily inadequate compared to the mother's phantasy of being the solving element of her internal pain. The failure in achieving maternal *rêverie* seems to be connected with the mother's pain of having a baby who does not correspond to her unconscious desire.

This unconscious desire was, in the cases of these women I will present, an element that made the therapeutic work, namely the possibility of giving up the illusion of omnipotence, particularly difficult. The latter was fed by the continuous recourse to reproductive technologies, associated with omnipotent desires, whereas the experience of painful losses, not only of a loved one but also – as in these cases – of the longed-for baby and the loss of the idea of an omnipotent fertility, requires a process of mourning. Relinquishing the idea of an omnipotent fertility became possible in the therapeutic work as the conflict over loss of fertility became more conscious – rather than being denied – thus allowing some steps to the mourning process to take place.

Illusion and illusional belief

Illusions can be used to protect oneself from the need to face the truth concerning limitations and the sense of helplessness in dealing with infertility. The desire for motherhood leads to using illusions to overcome frustrations and obstacles. We all need illusion to protect ourselves from the impact of our frightening internal and external reality. Without illusion, that is, the hope which sustains the possibility that things might get better, life would be unbearable.

Two theoretical concepts form the base of my reflections: on the one hand is Winnicott's concept of *omnipotent illusion* (1953) which implies the mother's capacity to adapt to the infant needs so that the infant 'feels like God', as well as her capacity to facilitate the process of disillusionment which is the fundamental experience for a *nascendi* self to begin to become a self.

On the other hand, there is Britton's concept of '*illusional belief*' (1998), a belief which cannot be relinquished even when invalidated by reality testing, whereas if subsequent experience and *knowledge* discredit a belief, it needs to be relinquished, and this requires a process of mourning.

According to Winnicott, the mother's attention and adaptation to the needs of the child allows him to live in the illusion that he could control her with omnipotence:

A subjective phenomenon develops in the baby, which we call the mother's breast. The mother places the actual breast there where the infant is ready to create, and at the right moment [...] This is an important experience in the construction of the self, along with the gradual process of disillusionment, which can only occur if the mother has been capable of providing a sufficient experience of illusion.

(1953, p. 11–13)

Experiencing illusion is therefore necessary and represents for Winnicott a third area of the mind on which we depend in order to 'live creatively': without illusion there would be no art, no creativity, no literature. If things go well in this gradual disillusionment process, the stage is set for the frustrations that we gather together under the word weaning; but it should be remembered that when we talk about the phenomena (which Klein, in 1940, has specifically illuminated in her concept of the depressive position) that cluster around weaning we are assuming the underlying process, the process by which opportunity for illusion and gradual disillusionment is provided (1971, p. 13).

In describing intrauterine life, Ferenczi defines it as "subservient only to pleasure" and adds that the foetus "must get from its existence the impression that it is in fact omnipotent. For what is omnipotence? The feeling that one has all that wants, and that one has nothing left to wish for" (Ferenczi, [1913] 1994, p. 218–219). Klein also recognizes the value of illusion and of an ideal breast, which:

In its good aspect is the prototype of maternal goodness, inexhaustible patience and generosity, as well as of creativeness. It is these phantasies and instinctual needs that so enrich the primal object that it remains the foundation for hope, trust and belief in goodness.

([1957] 1997, p. 180)

Klein considers this period of illusion to favour development; the child enjoys illusions in order to explore new worlds until he or she is strong enough to integrate the two sides of the split – gratifying and frustrating – into a picture of the mother as she really is.

The meaning of illusion and its relationship with reality had already been explored by Freud, who argued that a belief can become an illusion "when a wish-fulfilment is a prominent factor in its motivation, and in doing so we disregard its relations to reality, just as the illusion itself sets no store by verification" ([1927] 1966, p. 31). With regard to the difficulties of letting go of an illusion, Britton describes the difference between belief and knowledge, and argues that beliefs require 'reality testing' to become knowledge: "If subsequent experience and knowledge discredit a belief, it needs to be relinquished; this requires a process of mourning if it is an important or precious belief" (Britton, 1998, p. 14).

At the origin of the patients' belief, there seems to be the presence of a particularly catastrophic Oedipal configuration in which they could not experience a 'triangular space' (Britton, Feldman & O'Shaughnessy, 1989) through which it is possible to acknowledge the link that joins the two parents and which contains all the potential relationships between them and with their child. It is through the mourning for the lost exclusive relationship between mother and child that one can realise that the Oedipal triangle does not mark the end of a relationship but just the end of an idea-illusion.

Through clinical material I will illustrate the patients' inability to give up an *illusional belief* and move to disillusionment and knowledge, and how they felt constantly and repeatedly compelled to overcome limits in the pursuit of this goal. Such a belief cannot be relinquished even when invalidated by reality testing, which would imply several elements which should restrain this desire, such as an evaluation of the woman's age and fertility or the absence of a partner willing to have a child, as well as the fact of having one or several children already.

In their treatment, my patients showed an inability to give up the belief of their fertility and work through the loss, in the deepest and most radical sense of the word. They had a pressing and overwhelming desire to achieve pregnancy with assisted reproductive technology. Despite the differences in their individual histories, these women shared several significant characteristics. First, they had all previously given birth to one or more children with ART after complex vicissitudes; second, all of them were relatively old and had disregarded medical advice against embarking on a second or third pregnancy; and, lastly, their partners were relegated to the background or even marginalized with respect to their choice of conceiving again. Another common aspect in my clinical experience is that these mothers asked me for a consultation not because they were under distress, but following the advice of professionals such as gynaecologists, paediatricians, or teachers who were worried about the difficulties in their children's mental and emotional development. Although the mothers had resolutely striven and suffered for so long to give birth to their children, they seemed to have little emotional attunement to their offspring. Their communications with their children were apparently characterized by some difficulty with maternal *rêverie* and a failure to provide adequate containment (Bion, 1959; 1962).

I will describe two brief clinical illustrations: a prolonged consultation with a 45-year-old mother and her 18-month-old baby and a psychotherapy with a 47-year-old mother of a child aged three.

First clinical illustration

The first patient – Gloria – aged 45, is the youngest of three siblings, whose parents separated when she was 12. Gloria is referred to me by her children's paediatrician because of her relationship with one of her two 18-month-old twins, the boy. During the periodic check-ups, the paediatrician notices in Gloria a difficulty "tolerating" the little boy, who has very troubled sleep patterns.

Gloria is a pleasant but very neglected woman and when I meet her, I am struck by the low, monotonous, and colourless tone of her voice. In the first meetings, she mostly talks about the painful account of her conceptions and the illness of her husband, a successful manager who, after only one year of marriage, was diagnosed with testicular cancer. This caused him to undergo a series of surgical interventions, chemotherapy cycles and check-ups that naturally compromised his fertility.

For this reason, all their three children were born thanks to her husband's sperm that had been collected and frozen before the surgical interventions. After the birth of their first child – Luca, seven years old at the moment of the consultation – a long and fruitless pursuit of their second pregnancy began, characterized by several attempts, hopes and failures, of which Gloria underlines more than once the physical strain, the pain of disappointments, and her determination to achieve this goal despite the opposing medical advice, because her oocytes "have aged prematurely". After five years, the couple decided to resort to egg donation, which she describes as an emotionally irrelevant fact and dismisses in a few words: "For me it is not a problem and I obviously keep the secret ...".

In talking about the twin pregnancy and delivery, Gloria's account becomes emotionally compelling once again. The final particularly demanding four months, the extremely difficult delivery, marked by the anxiety about a potential asphyxia of the newborns, the twins' prematurity, a severe haemorrhage and, on top of that, the concern about Luca who, already troubled from seeing his mother transformed by the pregnancy, found her "swollen and yellow" in the hospital so much as she looked "dead". Hearing how, on that occasion and in the following months, the patient felt she had nobody to help her was striking, and when I put her loneliness feeling into words, she said that her mother's presence was useless, because "she is an anxious and depressed woman".

Gloria had always felt like the daughter who had to support her mother within an "unhappy family". Her memories convey to me the image of an unseen girl with a depressed mother "who wore a headband and moped up the hallway in the morning" while she and her two brothers got ready to go to school. On the other hand, after the separation her father had taken no interest in the children, so much so that her mother did not want him to be even mentioned. Her helplessness and deep resentment still vibrate in the tone of her narrative. As a young woman, she tried to leave home by enrolling in an university far from home.

Paradoxically, Gloria's different attempts to get away from her family of origin and to disidentify from a lifeless maternal image failed and made her feel as a depressed and neglected woman, with her husband telling her that after the twin pregnancy she has become "too ugly to be looked at". Like she did in her own childhood, the firstborn 7-year-old son seems to have taken a supporting function in the family, regretting and apologising for "not being able to be of more help with the twins".

At a countertransference level, Gloria conveyed to me a deep need to communicate her profound disappointment and resentment, but at the same time she did not seem to expect any help and understanding from me. Indeed, her way of talking showed rather her wish to tell me the answers she had already found for herself or to explain things that she had already worked through on her own. I found myself wondering what originated this insistence to pursue the objective of a twin pregnancy with egg donor insemination at that age, when she already had a child. We can hypothesize some competition with her mother who had three children, besides the necessity to deny her husband's and her own infertility, to deny her husband's estrangement and her own age-ing. But it seemed to me that what drove Gloria was something more radical and inalienable, that is, an absolute need associated with the necessity to give life to a dead Oedipal couple and to a dead baby girl/self by giving birth to a living child. But the living child she seemed to be needing was not the child that she found herself carrying in her arms.

Gloria comes with John, 18-months-old. I am struck that he doesn't look like his mother at all. He explores my consulting room, but he seems to be held back by the need to reassure himself about his mother's presence not through her gaze, that he never seeks, but rather through physical contact. She always describes John as the difficult child in the couple of the twins and admits her partiality for Maria. John has never slept, has been breast fed for 13 months, has not separated from the breast easily (and he tends to seek it even now), seems never to relax, and calms down only when he is held.

His sister is the very opposite: she has been breast fed for four months, is calm, easy-going, and has found her development pace in a smooth and natu-ral way. Regarding this difference, I wonder what Maria might have felt in seeing her little brother being breast fed for almost one more year after she had been weaned.

While the mother turns her attention and speaks to me, John – who is half asleep in his mother's lap at first – wakes up, gets down, finds a little toy van with an open door. Then he turns to the curtain to see what stands behind it. During these moves he loses his balance and hits his head but does not com-plain. I comment on his curiosity and that he seems to be looking for a safe place. His mother does not intervene in the exchange between me and John and does not notice neither the words I address to him nor his sweet smile.

John is dealing with being confirmed and looked at. He never looks at his mother and rather seeks physical contact, which however does not satisfy him. He complains because he receives what he does not want and wants what he does not receive. John's sleep problems soon improve and after four sessions Gloria continues to come. In the meantime, she and her mother's relationship improves and they are going to spend the holidays all together. Gloria feels, for the first time, that she can receive support and she becomes able to ask for help.

The period of our summer holiday separation becomes even longer because Gloria has an accident with her scooter, and we meet up again later in autumn. The session is intense and filled with the pain connected to her health condi-tions and an increasingly deeper marital crisis. "It may seem a heresy – she confesses – but in difficult times I have asked myself 'Why did I do that?' I had a wonderful child. Who forced me to do it and find myself in choppy waters, to lacerate and tear myself apart?" I am deeply struck by her utterance that reveals some doubt and depressive feelings. It seems to express the impediment and the terror to abandon the power, to violate the law: a blasphemy. The analytic encounter makes Gloria feel the need to go through the process of mourning a part of herself, which has never experienced the mirroring and containing maternal function and has cast a very threatening doubt on her engrained belief. This allows her to face her emotional truth.

Second clinical illustration

Elena is referred to me by her gynaecologist, who is also a family friend. He is worried about her insistence in asking him to help her have a third pregnancy. Elena is a 47-year-old woman, already the mother of a 7-year-old girl, Clara, and a 3-year-old boy, Edward, both born with ART. Her husband is 20 years older and has "lazy sperms" which, together with the woman's reduced ovarian reserve, seems to be the main obstacle to their ability to procreate. So, they decided to resort to ART and Clara was born. To fulfil Elena's desire to have a second child, this first birth was followed by long years of further attempts: the woman underwent several treatments/stimulations, going through expectations, disappointments, failures and two miscarriages. After four years, Edward was born. The physical and emotional pain and the effort implied take up much space in our first session and Elena sums up her mood during those long years with a few meaningful words: "It had become a fixed idea. I wanted another child, and I was detached from everything!" However, Elena tells me almost embarrassed that after Edward's birth: "Then … how shall I say … I was left with a bitter taste … as if I had surrendered and said: 'Is that enough?'". "Surrender to what?", I ask. "I don't know …", she replies.

In fact, Elena is thinking about getting pregnant again, talking insistently with her gynaecologist who, considering that the woman's ovarian reserve is not sufficient, notices her insistence with alarm. At a countertransference level, on the one hand Elena seems to be willing to talk about herself and share her painful feelings but, on the other, she admits: "It is not easy to come here …. Perhaps it may sound presumptuous, but I'm doing a lot of self-analysis". Struck by this debut, I wonder to what extent the patient can feel our work as being imposed by the gynaecologist, and often the analyst entails the risk of becoming, in the transference, a maternal object which opposes fertility (Quagliata, 2010). Elena expresses this by saying: "Anyway, even if I came for a whole year, you would not be able to change my mind".

Elena's intense loneliness, like Gloria's, would emerge again painfully when the memories of her parental couple come to light. Her parents had always ignored each other; she had a strict and rigid father and a self-absorbed mother, with whom she had never shared any intimacy or tenderness and to whom she had not even talked about her artificial insemination.

When she speaks about her children, she almost seems to struggle to find the words and, like Gloria, she is able to talk about them mainly in dichotomous terms: Clara, her eldest daughter, is calm and reflective, whereas Edward has always been a very vivacious boy with sleep problems. The nursery teachers have defined him as a hyperactive and unsocial child. When she was trying to achieve her second pregnancy, she was convinced that she would have a "second Clara", but then she realised that this was not the case.

Elena's appearance, an attractive and elegant woman, is always striking because of the dark rings under her eyes, but when she talks about babies her face seems to light up. Over time, Elena seems to decide she wants to spend more time with her children and enjoy what she has. I wonder if experiencing a chance to recover and meet the needs of her internal child in the therapeutic relationship has mitigated her urge to have another baby to care for.

However, one day Elena cancels her following session and I do not see her anymore. The gynaecologist tells me that two weeks after our last meeting, she contacted him because she wanted to undertake another ART treatment. Faced with the refusal of the doctor, the woman aggressively revealed that she had already made an appointment with another centre for egg donor insemination.

I wonder to what extent, in Elena's mind, this insistence was supported by the *illusional belief* of triumphing over the experience of catastrophe. The 'fertility' of our work together – which allowed her to experience however briefly a new image of the parent-child couple – would question this belief and would require the need to mourn that loss.

Discussion

I have tried to reflect on some common aspects in these women that made them similarly fragile and problematic. The failure of maternal containment and *rêverie* prevented these patients from seeing their children's pain, which was evident in the eyes of those who referred them to me. Like in the mothers' childhood, the loneliness experienced in lacking maternal mirroring function (Winnicott, [1967] 2002) seems to reappear in the next generation. Perhaps it is for this reason that both children had sleep problems; but after a few sessions with their mothers, they were able to fall asleep more easily. We can assume that their difficulty was connected to the feeling of having to control and comfort their mother.

For Gloria and Elena, the desire for a child during pregnancy seemingly remained in the realm of omnipotence, and the 'other' could only be imagined. However, when the child became 'real', he was rejected; there wasn't a place for him in their mind.

The etymology of 'conception' is interesting. It comes from "*cum-capere*", that is, "to receive inside". These mothers lack a mental space where these beings can 'nest'. One wonders about the burden that the child, involved in the mother's illusion, bears unknowingly. Having to sustain the guilt – feeling necessarily inadequate compared to the mother's phantasy of his being the solving element of her internal pain – the child is forced to confront the pain of having not met his mother's desire. We therefore see the burden of the catastrophe, unmourned by the mother.

Psychoanalytic observation has shown that although these procedures may be successful, a woman's inability to deploy her procreative capacity undermines her self-image (Raphael-Leff, 2013). It constitutes a major traumatic mental event, and for some mothers it may represent a fear of loss of the very matrix of their identity, with the dramatic consequence that they feel devoid of significance.

Some authors (Apfel & Keylor, 2002) also suggest it may even lead to an experience that parallels the typical suffering of the terminally ill. In particular, the couple must work through a failure and confront the reality of having been unable to conceive and create life as their own parents did; that is to say, they must go through a mourning process (Pines, 1990).

In the therapeutic relationship, it appears clearly that the difficulty to mourn involves not only the loss of fertility and the miscarriages. When Gloria 'conceives' for the first time the idea that her life could have had another course, she expresses herself strongly by saying: "It might seem a blasphemy!". At the time of insight and deep understanding, a powerful confrontation with a super-ego, a phantasy/belief that cannot be challenged and that protects her from mourning, and the risk of a catastrophic loss seem to be triggered.

The recognition of an Oedipal situation represented by the meeting with the analyst – analyst/paediatrician or analyst/headmaster – implies the recognition of a need, which has been so dramatically disregarded, and the contact with painful feelings of depression that, in turn, prompt the mourning process. This is what, I think, seriously jeopardizes the involvement of these women in the therapeutic work. In fact, it is not only a matter of mourning and working through infertility and miscarriages, but also perceiving a disaster and the risk of disintegration, a catastrophic change. The compulsive need of going through fertility treatment can become a retreat, a defence that makes it more difficult to relinquish a belief which doesn't meet reality testing and to face the truth beneath the illusion.

We believe that women with infertility problems benefit from psychoanalytical psychotherapy in which they gradually discover an internal space – rather than a hole – and inner resources (Raphael-Leff, 1991), getting in touch with their resentfulness, guilt, helplessness and deprivation, as well as their inner creativity.

Conclusion

I tried to investigate some links that seem to underlie the compulsive search for motherhood in a certain kind of female patients, and the difficulties of abandoning the *illusional belief* rooted in their early child development, when they experienced a particular failure in dealing with the Oedipal situation. Reality testing requires the presence of a triangular psychic space with a third position from which the subjective self can be observed having a relationship with the idea: the holder of a belief can therefore accept the possibility of it being untrue.

In this respect, these women had little desire to talk about their relationship with their partners as if they did not want to think about the events that had led to the dismantling of an *illusional belief* about the couple. The difficulties in the couple relationship were hard to explore as well as the relegation of the patients' husbands, who did not want to be involved in the treatment, even though the difficulty also originated in the couple's failure to mourn their fertility.

Such marginalization was also expressed in the therapeutic relationship, in which they relegated the therapist: "I am doing self-analysis". Analyst and patient could not become a creative couple. There was a threat of continuing the therapeutic work and thus transforming belief into knowledge. Being able to continue the treatment was affected by the fact that the request for help did not come from the women themselves, as they were not aware of the problem and therefore were not as motivated as they might have been.

I reflected on the failure of empathic mirroring in the relationship these patients had with their mothers, who were too caught up in their own wounds, as well as their children's emotional and behavioral difficulties through the transgenerational repetition of trauma. The difficulty of establishing a bond with the real child thus seems to be rooted in my patients in the presence of the previously lost children in the mother's mind, and the impossibility of having a space for the new child. Furthermore, it was also rooted in the need to bring into the world a self deprived of an understanding and loving gaze from a depressed mother (Green, 1999), whom they were unable to revitalize and with whom the patients ended up feeling identified. All the children had quite significant sleep problems that disappeared within a few weeks after their mothers began treatment. This could be thought of as maternal phantasies of dead babies that are passed on in the fears of the children.

I therefore would like to point out the importance of early intervention and cooperation with other professionals in treating these vulnerable mothers, as well as the technical issues concerning interpretation and countertransference difficulties. Several authors have addressed feelings of helplessness and frustration resulting from many of these women's refusal to engage in the analytic work (Faure-Pragier, 1993).

Loss and mourning, Oedipal configuration and *illusional belief* are all relevant, in my opinion, to the subject's dimension of infertility and birth and the whole perinatal (and later) period. The capacity to give up the illusion of omnipotent fertility is a crucial factor. "Childless women can hold a creative maternal function, placing themselves within a symbolic creative couple, whereupon mothers with many children can experience significant difficulties in relation to their own capacity to be and to feel authentically creative" (Raphael-Leff, 2000, p. 19–20).

In my reflection on the insistence with which some women pursue a pregnancy with ART, and given the difficulties they encounter in the relationship with their children, I argue that the difficulty to process the mourning for an *illusional belief* is what seems to drive these women to insist in their desire to procreate. The *illusional belief* is that of being able, through procreation, to exercise power over the experience of loss, not just on their lack of fertility and previous miscarriages, but on becoming aware that a loss did happen – that of not having been a child conceived in the mind and in the gaze of two parents who failed in creating an Oedipal triangulation. This belief gives these women life and makes them feel real, but it is an external solution to an internal problem and is doomed to fail. Rather than being recognized and mourned, the loss is reproduced in some form of repetition compulsion: manically recreating rather than mourning. The child created in intense loneliness, the concrete result of an insistent pursuit, is not what the mothers would have wanted. Perhaps also being male babies played a role in this failure because it made them even more distant from a re-edition of themselves.

One of the major difficulties for the analyst is that in moving from a position of solidarity, support and mirroring, the analyst is afraid of embodying the image of a mother who prohibits fertility and the paths which lead to it, "an image that is present in all of us, and all the more so in a woman with fertility problems" (Goretti, 2012, p. 1163). Yet clinical experience shows that the search for meaning and unconscious motivation – the leaven of psychoanalytic observation and listening –, when accompanied by respect for the surprising diversity of forms of psychic reality, will enable these patients to face the truth beneath the *illusional belief* and to work through a process of mourning, thus achieving a new fertile meeting with their own thoughts and minds.

Starting from the idea that the generative function is not necessarily connected to motherhood, the capacity to bring to life can be thought of, in my opinion, as the result of an introjection of the creative Oedipal couple and an identification with a 'generative mother'. In my view (Quagliata, 2022), we could consider fertility as the human ability to begin something new, to start a new process; something close to the category of "natality" mentioned by Arendt (1958) as the ability to introduce a new beginning in time, which is rooted in the human condition of being born.

Note

1 The maternal capacity of containment also depends on the existence of sufficient support in the external reality (partner, family) and on the number of other demands that can be borne (financial, domestic) and affect her mental space and energy.

References

Apfel, R. & Keylor, G. (2002). Psychoanalysis and infertility. *International Journal of Psychoanalysis*. 83: 85–104.
Arendt, H. (1958). *The human condition*. University of Chicago Press.
Bion, W. ([1959] 1967). Attacks on linking. In *Second thoughts* (pp. 93–109). Maresfield.
Bion, W. (1962). *Learning from experience*. Karnac.

Britton, R., Feldman, M. & O'Shaughnessy, E. (1989). *The oedipus complex today.* Karnac.

Britton, R. (1998). *Belief and imagination.* Routledge.

Faure-Pragier ([1913] 1993). L'insoutenable neutralité du psychanalyste face à la bio-éthique. *Revue Française de Psychanalyse,* 4: 1229–1246.

Ferenczi, S. ([1913] 1994). Stages of development of the sense of reality. In *First contributions to psychoanalysis* (pp. 213–239). Hogarth Press.

Freud, S. ([1927] 1966). The future of an illusion. In *Standard editions, volume XXI* (p. 1–58). Hogarth Press.

Garland (1988). *Understanding trauma: A psychoanalytical approach.* Karnac.

Goretti, G. (2012). On procreating today. *International Journal of Psychoanalysis,* 92: 1153–1173. DOI: 10.1111/j.1745-8315.2012.00640.x

Green, A. (1999). *The dead mother.* Routledge.

Klein, M. ([1957] 1997). Envy and gratitude. In *Envy and gratitude and other works* (p. 176–235). Vintage.

Klein, M. ([1940] 1998). Mourning and its relation to the manic-depressive states. In *Love, guilt and reparation and other works* (pp. 344–369). Hogarth Press.

Pines D. (1990). Pregnancy, miscarriage and abortion. A psychoanalytic perspective. *International Journal of Psychoanalysis,* 71: 301–307.

Quagliata (2010). *Becoming parents and overcoming obstacles.* Routledge.

Quagliata (2022). Discussion paper at the panel 'Idealization of motherhood'. In EPF Congress '*Ideals*', Vienna, March 24 to 26, 2022.

Raphael-Leff, J. (1991). *Psychological processes of childbearing.* Chapman and Hall.

Raphael-Leff, J. (2000). *Spilt milk: Perinatal loss & breakdown.* The Institute of Psychoanalysis.

Raphael-Leff, J. (2003). *Parent infant psychodynamics: Wild things, mirrors and ghosts.* Routledge.

Raphael-Leff, J. (2007). Femininity and its unconscious 'shadows': Gender and generative identity in the age of biotechnology. *British Journal of Psychotherapy,* 23: 497–515.

Raphael-Leff, J. (2013). *Pregnancy: The inside story.* Routledge.

Reid, M. (2003). Born in the shadow of death. *Journal of Child Psychotherapy,* 29: 207–226.

Winnicott, D. (1953). Transitional object and transitional phenomena: A study of the first not me possession. *International Journal of Psychoanalysis,* 34: 89–97.

Winnicott, D. (1971). *Playing and reality.* Penguin Books.

Winnicott, D. ([1967] 2002). Mirror-role of mother and child development. In J. Raphael-Leff (Ed.). *Parent-infant psychodynamics* (pp. 14–21). Routledge.

Chapter 4

"The Empty Cradle"

Envy, shame, and shaming in infertility

Melis Tanik Sivri

Introduction

The title of this chapter, "The Empty Cradle", refers to feelings of loss and mourning experienced during the processes involving the use of assisted reproductive techniques (ART), on the one hand, and to the eagerly awaited baby and the hope for it, on the other. As a metaphor, it is inspired by the author's clinical experiences working with women who resort to ART, as well as an old Turkish film with the same title, engraved in the collective memory of Turkish culture. The aim of this chapter, however, is to reflect on the dynamics of envy and shame which tend to emerge in and between women in cases of infertility, illustrated by the movie "The Empty Cradle".

Shame is a painful emotion which stems from a sense of failure to live up to one's image of a fertile woman and an ideal mother in the mind of women that needs to be worked through during the analytic treatment of infertility and ART. Overt feelings of shame may also be encountered as a defense against feelings of envy and jealousy towards other women who already have babies or who are perceived as having such a potential. What I would like to discuss in this chapter, however, is not only the feelings of envy and internal shame which may emerge in women experiencing infertility, but the external shaming to which they may be subjected to by other women, as portrayed in the film "The Empty Cradle". One should bear in mind that there is also a cultural aspect to this, given that Turkey is one of the countries where shaming is used by some parents as a childrearing technique and a tool for controlling the bodies and regulating the behaviors of little girls from very early on. From a psychoanalytic perspective, however, I believe it is related to the complexities of the mother-daughter relationship originating from the "sense of sameness" that is shared by the mother-daughter dyad.

As is well known, "the sense of sameness" experienced by the mother-daughter dyad due to having the same sexed body makes separation a challenging process for women. This process is, more often than not, considered from the point of view of the daughter – the child of the mother. However, mothers may also have different levels of difficulties in separating from their

DOI: 10.4324/9781032693446-4

daughters, especially those who have not worked through their pre-Oedipal and Oedipal conflicts sufficiently. Keeping in mind the mutual difficulties – albeit in different intensities and in different levels – experienced by both daughters and mothers, who share a sense of "sameness" yet are not "identical", may further our understanding regarding the complexities of the mother–daughter relationships and the conflicts which arise specifically in woman-to-woman relationships. It is possible that a woman's desire and her attempts to have a child, or indeed pregnancy itself, may trigger infantile phantasies about the maternal body and the related female castration anxieties as well as a heightened investment in the woman's body not only in her mind, but in the mind of the other women around her as well. The woman's body becomes a locus for curiosity and external projections of idealization and admiration, on the one hand; envy, competition, rivalry and fear, on the other. Following this line of thought may be helpful in illuminating the dynamics of envy and shame felt by women who experience infertility as well as the external shaming imposed upon them by other women, as can be observed in the film "The Empty Cradle".

"The Empty Cradle": The film

"The Empty Cradle" is a Turkish film based on a theater play, written by the famous Turkish writer and poet Necati Cumali in 1949, a classic work compiled from the folk tales in the Aegean region, transmitted orally from one generation to the next. In this play, Cumali takes the great Greek tragedy poets Sophocles and Euripides as his model. He uses folkloric elements in order to depict the lives of people oppressed under the pressure of honor and traditions in the rural life of Western Anatolia (Temel, 2007). Some of these folkloric elements which are present in the play linked to well-established traditions are beliefs around infertility, second wives, bad luck, fortune telling and evil eye (Savaş, 2010). In the overall corpus of the Turkish folk tales, one encounters the theme of infertility in 48 tales, going up to 123 with some variations on the theme (Cemiloglu, 1999). The story of "The Empty Cradle", however, has become one of the best-known tales thanks to Necati Cumali's play and the subsequent production of the movie with the same title.

The "Empty Cradle" tells the story of Fatma, a lowlander, who marries Ali, a nomadic landlord, despite the objections of the families on both sides. The film depicts the emotional struggles that Fatma endures during the seven years she is unable to get pregnant. It's imperative for Fatma to have a baby, especially a boy, for the continuation of the generation of Ali's family. Fatma is almost shunned from the community while Ali's mother and paternal uncle try to convince Ali to get a second wife. Ali fights vigorously against social pressure and just as he is finally giving in, Fatma gets pregnant. After a while, Murat[1] is born. The newborn brings great joy to the family and their extended circle.

Meanwhile, the men of the community are eager to start the migration without having to wait for the end of the puerperium. According to traditions, Fatma, being a lowlander, travels at the end of the migration queue, pulling a camel upon which her baby is placed in a cradle. Just as they start moving, they see an eagle flying in circles up in the sky which is believed to bring bad luck. Fatma strenuously walks at the very end, managing the camel while stopping at times to breastfeed her baby. Little by little the eagle approaches the cradle. As the scarf Fatma embroidered for Murat falls from the cradle onto the ground, she feels an excruciating pain in her heart. Feeling alarmed, she wants to check on Murat and realizes that the eagle has taken away her baby and all she sees is the sight of *the empty cradle*. Distraught with grief, Fatma embarks on a relentless struggle with the eagle which has devoured her baby. At the end of the film, she manages to catch the eagle with her bare hands but loses her balance. Fatma and the eagle fall off the cliff to their deaths as Ali watches them from afar. "The Empty Cradle", with its dramatic ending has left a deep and almost a traumatic imprint on the minds of many viewers from a certain generation in Turkey.

Infertility and shame

The desire for a baby is the product of the desire that couples have for each other. Alkolombre (2023) suggests that it is a product of the elaboration of an unconscious desire, unique to each subject, marked by pre-Oedipal and Oedipal conflicts. Becoming a parent requires a process of psychic preparation in which one reflects on their own identifications with their parents as well as working through the conflicts one experiences in relation to them. In Turkish culture however, as soon as couples get married, they face an expectation and sometimes even pressure from their families and close circles to have a child. Having a child is considered an important milestone in the couple's life and a symbol of social status. Women's bodies, being the locus of pregnancy, may be subjected to curious gazes from the outside as they try to detect a change, and at times are subjected to not particularly subtle remarks, leading to feelings of intrusion, discomfort, shame and inadequacy.

In "The Empty Cradle", Fatma, who is not able to get pregnant for seven years suffers from deep internal shame as well as shame imposed upon her from the community, especially from women. In the seventy years since this play has been written, there have been significant developments in the field of ART[2] and in how (childless) women are perceived in Turkish culture. With changing living conditions, some women have stepped out of their traditional roles, taking a more active place in the work force. Couples who marry later and decide to have children later than what was common in the past face not only societal pressure, but also time pressure. For women who feel this time pressure, conflicts arise between their desire to have a baby and their career aspirations. After the age of thirty-five, which is considered "advanced maternal age" for women, pregnancy carries various risks for the baby and fertility rapidly declines. With menopause, the fertility function completely disappears. Due to delayed pregnancies, side effects of contraceptive methods and urban-environmental factors, an increase in infertility and an increasing use of ART are observed globally (Raphael-Leff, 2014), including in Turkey.

Although the new developments in medicine and ART have lifted some of the stigma imposed on women in cases of infertility, in Turkey the play "The Empty Cradle" is still relevant nevertheless, in the sense that there is an undercurrent of self-blame and being blamed by others which lead to feelings of guilt and shame in women. A variously interpreted hadith by the Prophet Muhammad "Heaven lies beneath the feet of your mother" not only speaks to the importance given in Islam to children treating their mother with love and respect, but also to the strong influence of mothers in raising their children and thus the extent of idealization of motherhood. In rural areas, the couple's inability to conceive is still likely to result in a) finding women at fault for being childless despite medical evidence, b) divorce or c) a demand for a second wife.

Psychoanalytic literature reveals the existence of feelings of shame in couples who experience infertility (Zerbe, 2019; Siegel, 2017; Kramer & Steinberg, 2016; Freeman-Carroll, 2016; Vigneri & Carmody, 2012; Kremen, 2012; Kulish, 2011; Leon, 2010; Ehrensaft; 2008, 2000; Reenkola, 2005; Allison & Doria-Medina, 1999; Pines, 1990) some of which even link adoption-specific shame to the infertility of the adoptive parents (cited in Guittard, 2022; Wright, 2013, 2009; Balsam, 2011; Wade, 2010). Pines (1990) indicates that couples experience infertility as a failure that they cannot deny, which then leads to feelings of shame because they compare themselves to their friends who are able to have babies, as well as feelings of guilt since they are not able to give grandchildren to their parents for the continuation of the generation of the family. This in turn leads to trial periods, full of social and economic hardship, sometimes spreading over many years, in which women are exhausted both physically and emotionally while the relationship of the couple is affected adversely. These chronic trials bring about further feelings of shame and failure and result in a gradual erosion in confidence with respect to one's body-self and one's sexual self (Munschauer, 1997).

Rosen (2002) argues that women are more likely than men to take personal responsibility for the couple's inability to conceive. Childbearing is often perceived as women fulfilling their traditional role (Notman, 2011) and attaining their ego ideal of a maternal self (Pines, 1990). Interestingly, Berg and Wilson (1990; as cited in Keylor and Apfel, 2010) indicate that even when men are found to be responsible for infertility, women still express shame, guilt and self-blame. These authors argue that this may be partly due to the fact that women would like to protect men from injury. Based on clinical experience, I would like to suggest that this is also the case when women would like to protect men from their own disappointment and rage over their partner experiencing infertility, as well as deal with feelings of guilt emerging from their destructive phantasies and envy towards men's potency and virility. Self-blame can also be understood in association with women's feelings of omnipotence or their partial identification with the aggressor – patriarchal views prevalent in a culture which regards women as inferior.

Kramer and Steinberg (2016) discuss the enduring impact of shame when a baby is conceived through ART and must start life in the NICU. The mothers not only feel shame about the failure to conceive without assistance and the shame of having their "bodies poked and prodded, estrogen and progesterone levels measured" (p. 27), but also shame over the fact that even after the baby is born, assistance is needed in order to keep him alive or in one mother's case shame over not having enough milk for the baby. The authors talk about how couples who have kept their fertility treatments as a secret may now choose to keep the birth a secret, too, which leads to feelings of shame and alienation.

A case in the article is also worth mentioning where the intolerant reactions of the nurses and the patient's mother point to an inability to understand the grief of the patient who previously had stillborn twins and her current feelings of shame and inadequacy. This brings us to "The Empty Cradle", where women's intolerance towards and ostracization of Fatma by labeling her as an ominous figure is remarkable. How can we understand the deep sense of internal shame that Fatma experiences, as well as the intolerance and shaming to which she is subjected by other women? And how is it that Fatma is being represented as an ominous figure (uğursuz) infecting those around her with infertility in the mind of the women in the community?

Mothers and daughters: separation, envy, and shame

The relationship between mothers and daughters is complex. Freud ([1926] 1959), in *The Question of Lay Analysis*, states: "We know less about the sexual life of little girls than of boys. But we need not feel ashamed of this distinction; after all, the sexual life of adult women is a 'dark continent' for psychology" (p. 212). Despite the blindspots inherent in his theory of phallic monism (Chasseguet Smirgel, 1976), Freud ([1931] 1964) made an important discovery which became a departure point for the subsequent female analysts: that is the importance of the little girl's pre-Oedipal attachment to the mother in the development of female sexuality. Freud (1931) was struck that behind the strong attachment that the little girl has established with the father during the Oedipus phase, there lies the little girl's intense ambivalent attachment towards the mother. Further, to his surprise, he found out that this attachment persists into the fifth year of the little girl and that perhaps in many women it never fails to exist which makes it impossible for a change in the love object from mother to father. Kristeva (as cited in Perelberg, 2017), in fact, argues that women are in the impossible position of wanting both their fathers and mothers to be in one and the same love object which leads to an inherent bisexuality in women.

Reenkola (2005) in "Female shame as an unconscious internal conflict" talks about gender-specific shame as the little girl moves away from symbiotic love to separate love as she changes her love object. She talks about the difficulty of the little girl in separating from her mother and becoming aware of her desire for the father. She suggests that the core of a woman's shame is determined by the disappointments and rejections from both love objects – mother and father. She further indicates that a woman's ego-ideal is of a bisexual nature and that the "female inner eye" assesses not only "sexual appeal and motherliness but also performance and phallic achievements" (p. 104), making one especially vulnerable to shame if their superego is severely critical.

Thus, one of the fundamental questions that has been dealt with since Freud is how the little girl, who has the same sexed body as the mother, turns away from the "sense of sameness" she shares with the mother to the father, while inheriting what is necessary to become a woman and a mother. In case of differentiation, this "sense of sameness" sometimes leads to a fear of annihilation which women may try to defend themselves by resorting to masculinity complex or homosexuality, fall into melancholic depression, and/or develop bodily symptoms (Perelberg, 2017), including eating disorders due to an anxiety over the feminine sphere (Schaeffer, 2011) or perhaps involuntary childlessness.

The work of the feminine is a lifelong psychical journey. At different stages of life, as women experience significant bodily changes, they also need to re-examine and work through their relationship with their mother. This process begins with the birth of the girl and then continues through weaning, menstruation, first sexual intercourse, pregnancy, birth, puerperium, menopause and finally death. Every phase contains losses that must be mourned. Due to the generation gap, naturally, these different phases of life are not experienced by the mother and daughter concurrently. The daughter's desire to have a child is likely to emerge at a time when the mother is entering middle age, perhaps as she is getting closer to or experiencing menopause. For some mothers who are unable to grieve the loss of their youth and reproductive capabilities, seeing their daughters in the prime of their youth, getting ready to become mothers, may create unconscious feelings of envy and jealousy – especially since we live in an era where youth is glorified –, and in turn, feelings of guilt, shame and desire for reparation in the daughter.

One of the difficulties inherent in the separation process is the fact that the mother, besides being the first love object for the girl, is also the first object of identification that marks the girl's identity as a woman and a mother all her life. According to Guignard (2006), the little girl identifies with two psychic dimensions of the primary mother: a) the primary maternal sphere which represents mother's capacity for *rêverie* and containment; and b) the primary feminine sphere which represents mother's desire for the father and his penis. This is also the locus for the experience of absence and confrontation with the original fantasies of the primal scene and seduction. It's important to note that the "primary feminine sphere" facilitates the liberation from the mutual projective identification between mother and infant which takes place in the "primary maternal sphere". This liberation results in a sense of a loss of omnipotence as the child realizes that she is not the one and only object for the mother.

In girls, the mutual projective identification between mother and infant, prevalent in the primary maternal sphere, is from the beginning marked by an infinite set of mirror images. According to Guignard (2006), the mother's unconscious infantile dimension includes a representation of herself as a young girl and therefore both are experienced as being "the same". She contends that the endless mirror imaging between the mother's infantile dimension and that of her daughter puts the individuation process of the daughter in danger especially when the mother has a defective Oedipal structure, particularly if there are problems with paternal identification and cathexis of man-as-lover.

Godfrind (2001), on the other hand, suggests that the mother, from the beginning, has an original ambivalence towards her baby girl. The mother loves her daughter whom she perceives as the same, identical and similar which put them in an ideal state of intimacy, on the one hand; yet at the same time immediately perceives her to be a future rival which leads to an early distancing of the daughter from the mother. Perhaps it is this original ambivalence of the mother which lies in the archaic belief in Turkey that when a woman is pregnant with a girl, the baby takes away her mother's beauty (the little girl is out to steal and possess her mother's riches as in the Kleinian phantasy, even beginning from the womb); whereas if she is pregnant with a boy, the baby adds to her mother's beauty. On a similar note, it is believed that it is the evil eye of the mother which hurts the baby most, associated with the phantasized uncanny side of the mother.

Maternal body – feelings of envy, shame, and the uncanny

Freud ([1923] 1961) famously indicates that "The ego is first and foremost a bodily ego" (p. 26) and as such, phantasies regarding the mother's body are influential in the development of the little girl's unconscious representation of her own body. For the little girl, the maternal body, life-giving and death-dealing, is a source of admiration and identification on the one hand, envy and fear on the other. Is it possible that a woman's desire and attempts to have a child or pregnancy itself trigger infantile phantasies about the maternal body and related female castration anxieties not only in her mind, but also in the minds of other women around her?

As is well known, according to Freud ([1905] 1953), from the age of three the child is preoccupied with the question of "Where do babies come from?"[3] Often not getting a satisfactory answer from adults, he develops his own theories to answer this mysterious question. Contemplating on gender differences by comparing his own body with that of his mother, Little Hans gave clues to Freud about the child's feelings of jealousy and rivalry towards the same-sex parent, love for the opposite-sex parent, parental sexuality (primal scene), pregnancy and childbirth (Freud, [1909] 1955).

These are phantasies such as the mother being orally inseminated, the baby having been swallowed by the mother, the baby coming out of the mother's stomach by cutting through as in Little Red Riding Hood, or the mother giving birth anally. A representation of a terrifying and devouring mother persists in the infantile dimension of adult patients. This representation is, in fact, personified in the Turkish culture by the mythical figure – Alkarısı, similar to Lillith, who is believed to haunt women in the puerperal period in Anatolian folk belief, a product of the archaic fears and the reflection of women's aggression (Erten, 2017). In order to protect the woman who has just given birth, women in the family accompany her in her room for forty days, meanwhile she has to wear red or tie a red ribbon on the puerperal bed. Otherwise, it is believed that she is at risk of being suffocated by Alkarısı who will eat her internal organs and take away her baby. Thus, there seems to be a split between the "good" women in the family who will protect and care for the woman and will not leave her and the baby alone in the room as opposed to Alkarısı, a "bad" annihilating female figure who needs to be kept outside.

Freud ([1919] 1955) in his essay "The Uncanny", talks about the quote "Love is homesickness" (p. 231) and associates it with the original phantasy of returning back to the womb. He makes a connection between the maternal body and the uncanny; female genitalia as being the original home that we have once inhabited and which has ultimately become strange and foreign. Meltzer (1988) indicates that the "aesthetic conflict" results from feelings of uncanniness and suspicion that the mother's enigmatic interior creates in the baby on the one hand, and the admiration for the external beauty of the ordinary mother in the beginning of life on the other. Laplanche also argues that the maternal body carries enigmatic messages filled with the sexuality of the adult other that the infant perceives but gradually translates and makes sense of (Scarfone, 2014).

Klein (1932) considers childhood phantasies about the maternal body as the source of children's earliest anxieties. According to Klein, experiences of deprivation resulting from weaning lead to envious phantasies in children of both sexes of entering the mother's body and destroying its contents. According to the little girl, the mother's body is filled with all the riches she needs and wants to have, such as the father's penis, babies and feces. This fantasy also underlies the primitive origins of the Oedipus complex. The little girl unconsciously imagines her parents in a satisfying, endless sexual union while she remains outside of this couple. However, destroying the inside of the mother's body in phantasy creates in the little girl's psyche the fear that the mother will retaliate and rob and destroy her body. Most of all, she thinks that mother will harm her reproductive organs along with the potential babies inside. According to Klein, creativity stems from the child's desire to repair the inner mother destroyed in phantasy by envious attacks (Klein, 1929, 1940, 1945). But in some cases, when unconscious feelings of envy towards the inner mother and/or the parent couple are not softened by feelings of love and gratitude, reparation cannot occur.

Identification with a fertile and creative mother and a productive couple is hindered and difficulties may arise in conceiving a baby.

Anxieties regarding the enigmatic nature of the interior of the mother's body make it difficult for women to represent it, and therefore the interior of their own body. Guignard (2006) indicates that women can represent their wombs as differentiated from their mothers' wombs only after their first pregnancy, whereas Schaeffer (2011) states that women will experience this differentiation only when they lose their fertility with menopause. Based on her work with childless young women, Guignard (2006) indicates that when their mother suffers a gynecological problem, especially hysterectomy, these women experience not only fear of retaliation against their envious attacks on their mother's uterus, but they also experience it as a personal attack due to feelings of non-differentiation.

According to Balsam (1996), the focus of different theorists on the interior of the mother's body has led to "the female-to-female body comparison inherent in a woman's emotional growth" being overlooked. This is especially true for the pregnant body of the mother, which shows the potential and plasticity of the female body and is an important building block of body image (Yakeley, 2013). Balsam (1996) mentions that the pregnant body attracts the attention of everyone around and is the symbol of fertility and potency just like phallus, yet it is not given the same amount of attention in the literature. In order to get a full grasp of a woman's final body image, Balsam suggests:

> … to extend the territory of primary femininity to include from early on, a whole female-to-female body comparison which would then naturally include the small girl's fascination with the pregnant female body, the breasts, abdomen, buttocks, and all body parts including skin and hair as well as genitals.
>
> (1996, p. 402)

Early in her development, the little girl will most likely encounter the pregnant body of the mother, if not the pregnant body of the women in the family, and this will give her an outline of her future potential. As opposed to the invisibility of her genitalia, the swelling of the breasts and the belly in pregnancy are visible and these outer features will also trigger unconscious phantasies just like the invisible interior, which will then shape the development of the body image and femininity of the little girl. And in the case of infertility, feelings of shame and envy will arise out of a feeling of not being able to live up to the potential of one's body like the mother and the other women in the family.

"The Empty Cradle": feelings of envy, shame, and the uncanny

According to Reenkola (2005), a woman may feel that her worth is measured by pregnancy, which results in feelings of intense shame and sorrow in case of infertility. In "The Empty Cradle", the seven years that Fatma endures without a child are marked by internal and external shame, as well as feelings of sorrow and inadequacy. Although there is no medical examination which indicates that Fatma has infertility issues, she feels responsible for not having a child and tries to compensate by working very hard at home. Resigned to her fate, she expects her husband either to bring a second wife or send her back to her village. When women have difficulties conceiving, at times clinical experience shows that they may harbor feelings of idealization, envy, competition and rivalry towards women who may be represented in their minds as either an idealized fertile mother or an archaic retaliating and annihilating mother; or at times a generous, creative mother or a rivalrous Oedipal mother. The deep feelings of shame that Fatma experiences in "The Empty Cradle" may be considered to have two different sources: firstly originating from the narcissistic injury of not being able to conceive, fulfilling the potential of her body like her mother and the other women around her and living up to the cultural expectations and her ego ideal of becoming an "ideal mother", which is more apparent in the film, and secondly, as an unconscious defense against feelings of envy and jealousy which she may have towards these women whom she perceives as fertile and as rivals who can replace her any time.

Ali's mother is a significant character in the film, pressuring Ali from the start to get married to Elif from the nomadic community and give her grandchildren. Perhaps, this is a narcissistic desire on the part of the mother who perceives her future grandchild as a narcissistic extension of herself and perhaps even a phallus. While talking to a woman friend, she tells her that "there is no greater defect than infertility" and indicates that "their house is as gloomy as the house of the dead" – a castrated image of a woman associated with death. She believes that a woman has a voice and is respected only if she gives birth – idealization of motherhood. "Everyone despises the barren woman. God despised her and made her barren, why shouldn't the servant of God despise her?", she says. She constantly compares Fatma to Elif who has three children by then and often blatantly belittles her for not being able to conceive.

In the film, Fatma initially lives with her father and Ali lives with his mother. Both for Fatma and for Ali, this situation may be considered as a false Oedipal victory infused with feelings of guilt and shame. Although Ali's mother does not want him to get married to a lowlander, she goes to ask for permission from Fatma's father. Fatma's father rejects the proposal by humiliating Ali's mother. Fatma begs for forgiveness from Ali's mother and ends up eloping with Ali, leaving her father in shame. Thus, from the beginning Fatma and Ali's marriage is marked with feelings of guilt and shame, going against traditions and their parents' will. One wonders if their inability to conceive is a price they have to pay for this upheaval. By leaving her father behind, does Fatma own up to her desire of having a man of her own that she loves? Or is she leaving her father for a mother figure whom she has lost and to whom she is loyally attached with guilt? And what can we say about her desire for a baby? Is it stemming from the desire she feels for her husband? Or is it stemming from a desire to give a baby boy to a mother figure out of a wish for reparation by endowing her with a phallus?

Fatma is exposed to shaming and direct/indirect sarcastic remarks not only by her mother-in-law, but also by the women in the community. When Fatma helps a little girl who falls on the ground while playing, the mother of the girl immediately calls her daughter and tells her not to get close to "the ominous one". Later, while Fatma plays with a little boy, the boy tells her that he is afraid he will be jinxed and throws the beads that Fatma gave to him as a present. Fatma ends up praying to God for a child or else, for her life to be taken. She tells her only friend in the whole community, a woman friend: "I'm like a tree with a worm inside it! I'm drying up from within! No leaves, no flowers, no blossoms on my branches! Everyone runs away from me! Even children." It is interesting that she continues by saying that she would be fine with this situation if her husband was a shepherd and they were living alone, but what really kills her is the sullen faces and the sarcastic remarks of the community, especially her mother-in-law.

And when Fatma finally gets pregnant, although her mother-in-law changes her attitude towards Fatma in a positive light, the contempt of the women in the community, especially the contempt of Elif, her rival, continues, this time by denigrating Fatma on the basis that she cannot possibly give birth to a baby boy. We can understand Elif's attitude towards Fatma based on feelings of envy and competition. Ali, being the lord of the nomadic community, is considered a good catch as he is an attractive young man who holds a position of power in the community. Therefore, by choosing Fatma, a lowlander, as a wife, Ali must have created a lot of jealousy and envy among women, especially Elif. As I have mentioned before, in order for Fatma to have a say in the community she must have a baby boy for the continuation of Ali's family. Therefore, Elif is using shame as a tool to destroy Fatma, making her feel that she does not possess any valuable qualities as a person and that she does not deserve someone like Ali.

The external shaming by other women in "The Empty Cradle" may be considered as a derivative of the envy towards the maternal body or as a projection of an intolerable inadequate, infertile, castrated part of themselves that women want to get rid of. The woman's body, by becoming the container for such hostile projections, in turn gets to be represented as abject and uncanny – hence seen as being ominous and contaminating those around her with bad luck. Women then try to deal with their fear of retaliation stemming from their own hostility which is now embodied in the childless, "empty" body, by ostracization.

Conclusion

A woman's desire to have a baby may provide opportunities for "maternal transmission", for feelings of care and camaraderie as well as act as a fertile ground for the manifestation of conflictual feelings of envy, competition and rivalry between women. Reenkola (2021) points out the scarcity of discussion in the psychoanalytic literature regarding women's envy towards other women as these malignant feelings trigger shame and guilt. This chapter was an attempt to reflect on feelings of envy and shame which emerge in and between women in cases of infertility, as illustrated in the movie "The Empty Cradle".

The sense of sameness due to having the same sexed body makes it challenging for women to differentiate, at times leading to fears of annihilation and bodily symptoms, perhaps in some cases even contributing to involuntary childlessness. More often than not, the difficulties are being discussed from the point of view of the daughter. However, mothers too may have differing levels and intensities of difficulties with regards to separating from their daughters (especially if they have not worked through their pre-Oedipal and Oedipal conflicts sufficiently), which may add to the difficulties of the separation-individuation process of the daughter. This intersubjective perspective may be helpful in understanding the complex dynamics that emerge between mothers and daughters and in woman-to-woman relationships in general.

For the little girl, one of the difficulties inherent in the separation process is that the mother, besides being the first love object, is also the first object of identification. The ego is first and foremost a bodily ego and as is known, the little girl's unconscious representations of her own body are based on the phantasies regarding the maternal body. For the little girl, the maternal body, life-giving and death-dealing, is a source of admiration and identification, on the one hand; envy and anxiety, on the other. The author suggests that a woman's desire and attempts to have a child or pregnancy itself may trigger infantile phantasies about the maternal body and related female castration anxieties associated with it, as well as a heightened investment in the woman's body not only in her mind, but in the mind of the other women around her as well. The woman's body becomes a locus of curiosity and external projections of idealization and admiration on the one hand; envy, competition, rivalry and fear, on the other.

Shame is a painful emotion stemming from a sense of failure to live up to one's image of a fertile woman and an ideal mother in case of infertility and ART. Overt manifestation of shame may also appear as a defense against feelings of envy, inadequacy and competition towards other women who already have babies or are perceived as having such a potential. Cultural expectations regarding the place of women in society, idealization of motherhood and external shaming may exacerbate these feelings and result in women trying to handle their pain in isolation.

Psychoanalytic treatment makes it possible for women to work on these difficult-to-bear emotions in the containing presence of an other and mourn the loss in their minds of not only one's image of a fertile woman, but also the loss of the image of being a fertile couple, as well as the loss of the imaginary baby. It also provides an opportunity for women to work through their pre-Oedipal and Oedipal conflicts with their mother with a focus on infantile phantasies regarding the maternal body along with transgenerational transmission of possible actual traumatic experiences related with fertility, pregnancy and delivery, which ultimately paves the way for healthy feminine and maternal identification with the analyst/mother in transference.

In case of infertility, women find themselves at a crossroad in terms of whether they will resort to ART or not. Proceeding with ART confronts couples with complicated decisions along the way, one being the termination of the embryos, which deserve thinking through instead of taking immediate action. These decisions, although creating feelings of guilt and shame in women, also create the illusion of omnipotence, which seem to be the flip side of the loss of phallic power. Psychoanalytic treatment helps women faced with such complicated decisions to distinguish between the wish to become a mother (Weldon, 2006) and the wish to become pregnant (Amati Mehler, 2006), or in Alkolombre's terms (2023) "the desire for a child" versus "the passion for a child", preventing chronic trials leading to physical, emotional and financial exhaustion.

One final issue worth mentioning related with feelings of shame that women endure is feelings of terror and the uncanny felt as a consequence of a sense of having strayed from the natural course of pregnancy, resulting in the phantasy of a "monster baby" with the counterpart of a "monster mother". The representation of the monster baby, or women's fears of bringing an "abnormal" baby, "a freak" into the world, can be thought of in relation to the woman's phantasies of retaliation by the archaic mother and/or her feelings of guilt over her Oedipal desires for her father. These fears are intensified by the traumatic pregnancy and childbirth experiences of women in the family or of the woman herself. These feelings, which may contribute to postpartum depression and attachment difficulties, are addressed and elaborated in the treatment.

To conclude, psychoanalytic work is pregnant with possibilities that enable women to discover their potential, their creative and productive sides, their capacity for sublimation, their maternal functions which include not only infant care and child rearing but also caring for another being, manifested in acts of solidarity (Alizade, 2006), and transforming their destructive sides. Based on clinical experience, the author proposes that analysis, especially woman-to-woman analysis, provides an "analytic cradle" for women whereby they are able to work through and elaborate on their infantile phantasies, thoughts and feelings – including shame and envy – and mourn their losses, as well as the opportunity to identify with the feminine and the maternal aspects of the analyst through transference where it is crucial for the analyst to work through their own countertransference.[4] As such, the author suggests that by providing a space where complex, conflicting and difficult-to-bear emotions can be enacted and worked through, analytic work can have a supportive impact on women's psyche and the couple's relationship during their assisted reproductive journey.

Notes

1 A Turkish male name which means "wish".
2 Turkey is one of the countries where egg and sperm donation, as well as surrogacy, are considered illegal.

3 For Freud's thoughts on birth, see Tanik, M. (2008). "How did I come into this world?: Rebirth through Psychoanalysis". *Freud Talks*. Istanbul: Yapi Kredi Publications.

4 I had discussed this issue with respect to the pregnancy of the analyst in "Woman to woman analysis: The impact of the concrete presence of the analyst's body in the transmission of the feminine" (2019, EPF Conference, Madrid; unpublished paper) and also with respect to ART in "The stranger in the house" (2023, EPF Conference, Cannes; unpublished paper).

References

Alizade, M. (2006). *Motherhood in the twenty-first century*. Routledge.

Alkolombre, P. (2023). *The Desire and Passion for a Child. Psychoanalysis and Contemporary Reproductive Techniques*. Routledge.

Allison, G. & Doria-Medina, R. (1999). New reproductive techniques. *International Journal of Psychoanalysis*, 80: 163–166.

Amati Mehler, J. (2006). Artificial pregnancy. In A. M. Alizade (Ed.), *Motherhood in the Twenty-first Century* (pp. 35–44). Karnac.

Balsam, R. H. (1996). The pregnant mother and the body image of the daughter. *Journal of the American Psychoanalytic Association*, 44S (Supplement): 401–427.

Balsam, R. H. (2011). The quest for motherhood: When fertilization fails. *Psychoanalytic Inquiry*, 31: 392–403.

Cemiloglu, M. (1999). *Birth motif in folk tales. [Halk Hikayelerinde Doğum Motifi]*. VİPAŞ Publishing.

Chasseguet-Smirgel, J. (1976). Freud and female sexuality—the consideration of some blind spots in the exploration of the 'dark continent'. *International Journal of Psychoanalysis*, 57: 275–286.

Ehrensaft, D. (2000). Alternatives to the stork: Fatherhood fantasies in donor insemination families. *Studies in Gender and Sexuality*, 1: 371–397.

Ehrensaft, D. (2008). When baby makes three or four or more: Attachement, individuation, and identity in assisted-conception families. *Psychoanalytic Study of the Child*, 63: 3–23.

Erten, Y. (2017). The uncanny return. [Tekinsiz dönüş]. *Suret Psychocultural Analysis Journal*. İthaki Publishing.

Freeman-Carroll, N. (2016). The possibilities and pitfalls of talking about conception with donor egg: Why parents struggle and how clinicians can help. *Journal of Infant, Child & Adolescent Psychotherapy*, 15: 40–50.

Freud, S. ([1905] 1953). Three essays on the theory of sexuality. In *The Standard Edition of the Complete Psychological Works of Sigmund Freud, Volume VII* (pp. 123–246). Hogarth Press.

Freud, S. ([1909] 1955). Analysis of a phobia in a five-year-old boy. *The Standard Edition of the Complete Psychological Works of Sigmund Freud, Volume X* (pp. 1–150). Hogarth Press.

Freud, S. ([1919] 1955). The 'Uncanny'. In *The Standard Edition of the Complete Psychological Works of Sigmund Freud, Volume XVII* (pp. 217–256). Hogarth Press.

Freud, S. ([1923] 1961). The Ego and the id. In *The Standard Edition of the Complete Psychological Works of Sigmund Freud, Volume XIX* (pp. 189–210). Hogarth Press.

Freud, S. ([1926] 1959). The question of lay analysis. In *The Standard Edition of the Complete Psychological Works of Sigmund Freud, Volume XX* (pp. 177–258). Hogarth Press.

Freud, S. ([1931] 1964). Female sexuality. In *The Standard Edition of the Complete Psychological Works of Sigmund Freud, Volume XXI* (pp. 221–244). Hogarth Press.

Godfrind, J. (2001). *Comment la féminité vient aux femmes?* Presses Universitaires de France. [(Tr. L. Mete), 2014, *Kadınlık Kadınlara Nasıl Gelir?* Bağlam Publishing]

Guignard, F. (2006). Maternity and femininity: Sharing and splitting in the mother–daughter relationship. In A. M. Alizade (Ed.). *Motherhood in the Twenty-first Century*. (pp 101–116). Karnac.

Guittard, J. (2022). When the good object is also a thief: A memoir of adoption. *Journal of the American Psychoanalytic Association*, 70: 39–76.

Keylor, R. & Apfel, R. (2010). Male infertility: Integrating an old psychoanalytic story with the research literature. *Studies in Gender and Sexuality*, 11: 60–77.

Klein, M. (1929). Infantile anxiety-situations reflected in a work of art and in the creative impulse. *International Journal of Psychoanalysis*, 10: 436–443.

Klein, M. (1932). *The Psycho-Analysis of Children*. Hogarth.

Klein, M. (1940). Mourning and its relation to manic-depressive states. *International Journal of Psychoanalysis*, 21: 125–153.

Klein, M. (1945). The Oedipus complex in the light of early anxieties. *International Journal of Psychoanalysis*, 26: 11–33.

Kramer, S. & Steinberg, Z. (2016). In hope's shadow. Assisted reproductive technology and neonatal intensive care. *Journal of Infant, Child & Adolescent Psychotherapy*, 15: 26–39.

Kremen, A. (2012). Beyond conception: Recovering the creative couple after infertility. *Couple and Family Psychoanalysis*, 2: 80–92.

Kulish, N. (2011). On childlessness. *Psychoanalytic Inquiry*, 31: 350–365.

Leon, I. G. (2010). Understanding and treating infertility: Psychoanalytic considerations. *Journal of the American Academy of Psychoanalysis*, 38: 47–75.

Meltzer, D. & Harris Williams, M. (1988). *The Apprehension of Beauty: The Role of Aesthetic Conflict in Development*. Clunie Press.

Munschauer, C. A. (1997). Shame: The dark shadow of infertility. In M. R. Lansky & A. P. Morrison (Eds.). *The Widening Scope of Shame* (pp. 235–243). The Analytic Press.

Notman, M. T. (2011). Some thoughts about the psychological issues related to assisted reproductive technology. *Psychoanalytic Inquiry*, 31: 380–391.

Perelberg, R. (2017). Love and melancholia in the analysis of women by women. *International Journal of Psychoanalysis*, 98: 1533–1549.

Pines, D. (1990). Emotional aspects of infertility and its remedies. *International Journal of Psychoanalysis*, 71: 561–568.

Raphael-Leff, J. (2014). *Dark side of the womb*. Anna Freud Centre.

Reenkola, E. M. (2005). Female shame as an unconscious inner conflict. *Scandinavian Psychoanalytic Review*, 28: 101–109. DOI https://doi.org/10.1080/01062301.2005.10592765

Reenkola, E. M. (2021). Envy between women. *Scandinavian Psychoanalytic Review*, 44: 59–66. DOI https://doi.org/10.1080/01062301.2022.2137312

Rosen, A. (2002). Binewski's family: A primer for the psychoanalytic treatment of infertility patients. *Contemporary Psychoanalysis*, 38: 345–370.

Savaş, Y. (2010). *A study of the elements of folk literature and folk culture in the works of Necati Cumalı. [Necati Cumalı'nın Eserlerindeki Halk Edebiyatı ve Kültürü Unsurlarının İncelenmesi]*. Master's thesis. Konya: Selcuk University.

Scarfone, D. (2014). A brief introduction to the work of Jean Laplanche. *International Journal of Psychoanalysis*, 94: 545–566.

Schaeffer, J. (2011). *The universal refusal. Psychoanalytic exploration of the feminine sphere and its repudiation.* Karnac.

Siegel, R. (2017). "Where did I come from?" The impact of ART on families and psychotherapists. *Psychoanalytic Inquiry*, 37: 512–524.

Temel, T. (2007). *A study of the "women characters" in Necati Cumali's play.* [*Necati Cumalı'nın Oyunlarındaki 'Kadın Karakterler'in İncelenmesi*] Master's thesis. Erzurum: Ankara University.

Vigneri, M. & Carmody, C. (2012). Children who come in from the cold: On infertile women and the new frontiers in procreation. *The Italian Psychoanalytic Annual*, 6: 143–167.

Wade, J. (2010). The long gestation: Adoption as a developmental milestone. *Modern Psychoanalysis*, 35: 24–52.

Weldon, E. (2006). Why do you want to have a child? In A. M. Alizade (Ed.). *Motherhood in the Twenty-first Century* (pp. 62–75). Karnac.

Wright, J. L. (2009). The princess has to die: Representing rupture and grief in the narrative of adoption. *Psychoanalytic Study of the Child*, 64: 75–91.

Wright, J. L. (2013). Discussion of "Why didn't they keep me?": The search for belonging in the analysis of a four-year-old adopted child. *Psychoanalytic Inquiry*, 33: 345–350.

Yakeley, J. (2013). Seeing, mirroring, desiring: The impact of the analyst's pregnant body on the patient's body image. *International Journal of Psychoanalysis*, 94: 667–688.

Zerbe, K. (2019). The secret life of secrets: Deleterious psychosomatic effect on patient and analyst. *Journal of the American Psychoanalytic Association*, 67: 185–214.

Chapter 5

Reflections on the concept of "Passion for a Child"

Graciela Cardó Soria

Introduction

This chapter will discuss the concept of "Passion for a Child"[1] developed by Alkolombre (2008) from her work with women experiencing reproductive disorders. In the author's words, the passion for a child refers to "a particular destination of the desire for a child in women; (…) it is characterized by affective intensity within a narcissistic-passionate dimension" (Alkolombre, 2020, pp. 355).

Passion for a child is about an intense search, fixity and object dependence that borders on self-destructive limits. It represents the transformation of the desire for motherhood into a passion for motherhood that, although it drives from life, entails the risk of a traumatic melancholy (Alkolombre, 2008).

In fact, it comes with the suffering comprised in the ideal of motherhood that afflicts certain women. Another aspect that the author highlights is that the child becomes the unique object, so we stand in a sphere of narcissistic functioning, of primordial and dyadic bonds.

The passion for a child and its multiple outcomes, which represent a permanent presence in our lives, in culture and in our clinical practice, leave important marks. The feelings, decisions and practices involved in the attempt to conceive a child and its outcomes affect society in general: not only the couple going through that situation, but of course their future sons and daughters.

Currently, reproductive disorders are well known. It's not unusual to have listened to or even accompanied someone undergoing different ART procedures. In many cases, these procedures bring desires; in others, they bring feelings of passion that run through a psychopathological spectrum.

In my clinical practice, I have been able to meet women who, for various reasons and circumstances, have undergone multiple treatments either to get pregnant, to choose the sex of the baby or to freeze eggs. The physical and emotional pain and the high amounts of anxiety that are unleashed throughout the multiple procedures are invariant.

In many cases – if we think about the passion of a child – all this reflects obsessive management, as well as an alienation of one's own desire. Often it

DOI: 10.4324/9781032693446-5

corresponds more to what Alkolombre (2008) calls a desire for a child, and if that is the case, people attend procedures with less anxiety and psychological suffering and with more awareness of what the body experiences. But in some cases we find the passion for a child. The following sections are some associations and elaborations about this important concept. It should be emphasized that the focus on the following ideas will lie on the passion that is manifested towards pregnancy and fertilization processes.

First association: *Pinocchio*

I'd like to start my reflections with one of the many fairy tales that marked my childhood: *Pinocchio*. It was the first image that came to my mind about the concept of passion for a child: the child carved on pinewood who wanted to turn into a real child, the old carpenter who wanted a real son, the Blue Fairy that was capable of giving life, and the countless characters that filled this child's world. In hindsight, I wonder if Geppetto's desire for a son was not just a desire, but a passion; that feeling that is so close to suffering ("passio" in Latin), that led him to patiently suffer the humiliations that his son inflicted on him and that were sweetened by Disney.

Second association: *Artificial Intelligence*

My second association is a 2001 film titled *Artificial Intelligence*, directed by Steven Spielberg on a screenplay by Ian Watson, based on a 1969 short story written by Brian Aldiss. The rights were acquired by Stanley Kubrick in 1970, who eventually handed the story to Spielberg in 1995. The film starts by showing a couple devastated because their only son does not wake up from a coma, so they decide to buy a robot child named David, who has been programmed exclusively to love his parents. As is later understood, only suffering will come from this decision.

Third association: Social media

Now I present, as if they were clinical vignettes, some social media content that play a great role in the issues we are discussing, published by two Instagram influencers.

These women share on social media both their pain and their ideals, while going through ART procedures. Sometimes without any show of affection; others, the other way round. These are contemporary ways to transmit ideals, values and experiences which are usually brought by women who come to our practice. Any psychoanalyst could have some of them as his/her patients and could have heard any of their stories in the clinical settings. To take into account the information that we receive through these channels about these women's experiences, and to share such information, opens the doors to think about this important topic in terms of culture. It is indeed a frequent human situation, allowing us to think about the diverse and complex levels of the situation and their sufferings, pleasures, joys and illusions. In other words, everything that human existence is made up of.

Here are some examples of some phrases that are shared on Instagram:

* I think only people who are going through this can understand.
* Everybody remembers the date and time when their life broke: mine is a day like today, a year ago. On December 19, 2017, at about 8 p.m. we were going to the emergency room of HM Montepríncipe.
* Today more than ever I want to give voice to so many women whom they have tried to silence with a "don't complain", "don't cry", "it doesn't matter", "don't think about it", "don't talk about it".
* And finally, puncture day arrived ... and ..."wow, how many follicles"; "My god, look at those oocytes!", "It looks really good, kiddos!"...
* Insist, persist, resist and never desist

The intense desire that becomes passionate, mixed with pain and suffering, many times transformed into harangues, could be viewed as expressions of the concept of passion for a child. I also highlight the positive aspect of the use of social networks, in the sense that doing so many women feel less alone during these procedures and throughout pregnancy. However, often they are also samples of what we can understand as manic defenses against pain.

Passion, alienation, idealization

When faced with the intense emotions that these memories and associations bring to me, ideas from esteemed psychoanalysts such as Piera Aulagnier (1993), Chasseguet-Smirgel (2003) and Massimo Recalcati (2018) come to my rescue and help. These authors developed some ideas and concepts about the bond between mothers and children, talking about the mark of mothers' desire left on their future children. The powerful seal that maternal wishes impose on the psyche has consequences on the present and future of her offspring. The ideas of these psychoanalysts will contribute to the concept of passion for a child, as developed by Alkolombre (2008).

Geppetto and the parents who bought David would account for the destiny of pleasure studied by Aulagnier (1993): love, alienation and passion. We could consider also those who fall on the spectrum of the passion for a child – as the example of influencers – as suffering from the "illness of ideality" that Chasseguet-Smirgel (2003) reflects on.

These are mothers and fathers with their respective ghosts, desires and transgressions, which Recalcati (2018) describes in fine detail to explain plots of unconscious inheritance that are mixed with one another, accounting for a peculiar crystallization in the passion for a child mode.

I'd like to highlight that I prefer to talk about spectrum and configurations, as well as to use the gerund mode, since I think that the passion for a child is a *position* that settles in the human being, a *position* as Klein ([1935] 1998) understood it; made up of a type of anxiety, a way of relating to the object and corresponding defenses. Mental and body pain, constant frustrations, added to personal and family history, can lead a woman to place herself in that *position*.

Fiction precedes reality, but reality surpasses it. The speed of technological, medical and biological progress is changing the way we are born, the way we live and even the way we die. The most omnipotent and primitive fantasies, which were previously the exclusive domain of movies or novels, become a reality thanks to biotechnology, which, for the most part, has not yet been assimilated into shared social imaginaries, let alone processed.

Thus, science has been allowing women and men to freely choose to conceive and have children without necessarily going through sexual intercourse. We are witnessing the detachment of sex, in terms of pregnancy-purposed coitus, as well as of the desire for motherhood. In other words, the desire – sometimes passion – for a child is no longer totally linked to sexual desire towards the sexual partner; in some cases, the love for the offspring can show independence from the oedipal derivative, leading us, in the case of passion, to narcissistic areas. Today, it will no longer be Geppetto's Blue Fairy, or the company that manufactures robots, the creator of the child; it will be the doctors and biologists that handle sophisticated technologies who, in many cases, will fulfill the wishes of women who want to become mothers without going through the pregnancy process, or getting pregnant without having had sexual intercourse, with or without feelings of sexual desire towards the partner, or those of women who only want pregnancy, but not the child, amongst many other possible scenarios.

"The passion for a child" – as Alkolombre (2008) develops it – "appears in the clinic within the conjugal bond, as a problem that affects women and that has no equivalent in men" (p. 54).

We have data that contributes to the idea that the passion for a child pertains exclusively to women. A qualitative investigation revealed the way in which couples viewed and interrelated along the ART process. As if it were a sequel of the play *Yerma*, by Federico García Lorca, the findings showed that women experienced infertility as a catastrophic crack in their role, while men tended to view conception difficulties as disturbing, but not tragic. It was also very common for couples to view infertility as a female problem (Greil, Leitko, & Porter, 1988).

Patricia Alkolombre (2008) describes the destinies of the desire for a child, which metamorphoses into passion. According to this author, a passion can drive towards life, but it can also:

- turn into melancholy;
- turn into fury;
- reveal the pain and the imaginary whirlwind around ideas and affections towards the absent and missing object;

- contain the impulse of life;
- but also the abyss of nothingness, death;
- guarantee women's phantasmatic survival;
- bring constancy-perseverance into the search: something that never stops.

Thus, almost poetically, the author leads us to think about narcissistic times and areas linked to passion. In many occasions, more than the child, what is insistently charged as an idea-act-obsession-passion, is the fertilization process itself, what the woman's body experiences: for example, extraction of eggs, *in vitro* fertilization, implantation of fertilized eggs in the body, genetic diagnoses, inconceivable losses such as repeated miscarriages, unfinished mourning, announcements of possible pregnancies and other "terms" that account for these painful processes, as the Instagram posts showed. All these situations can produce regressions to what Melanie Klein ([1935] 1998) called the "paranoid-schizoid position", which I think would shape the passion for a child.

Therefore, what would the pursuing-attacking object be? The body itself that expresses its independence from the mind? The eggs, the doctor, the instruments, the hormones? The husband, the friends, social media? It is the pain that wraps the body of the woman in suffering and that through defensive mechanisms transforms desire into need and passion, reaching the realm of idealization and narcissism.

I think a new internal object with which the woman will relate emerges in this project: being pregnant. Would pregnancy cover up the failure by correcting injured narcissism and bodies? In some cases, yes. And then, pregnancy and motherhood take the place of the Ideal, showing what Chasseguet-Smirgel (2003) called *"the illness of ideality"*.

A possible route to understand the passion-illness of ideality is provided by Piera Aulagnier and her book *The destiny of pleasure* (1993), in which she discusses alienation, love and passion. For Aulagnier, these three states are the destinies that the pursuit of pleasure can impose on our thoughts and our lives. The object of the alienation-passion, as well as the alienating force, are characterized by satisfying the goals of both Eros and Thanatos, forming a temporary and precarious drive fusion; let's say that the child's fertilization-conception project crystallizes it.

Far away remains her Identificatory Project concept, which is totally opposite to the concept of narcissistic omnipotence. This project assumes the finitude and the pain involved in thinking; that is, recognizing and accepting reality, the fact of not being able to do everything. In these cases, the child-object, internal and external, real and imaginary, could be placed in the category of needed object, ideal object, persecutory object, consoling object, healing object, redemptive and savior object.

In many cases we can assume that there is a strong charge-cathexis in the child, assisted fertilization, pregnancy and parenting project. However, when narcissistic regressions occur, everything but a project is left; we witness a compulsive repetition of a series of attempts and procedures. Piera Aulagnier (1993) affirms that nothing remains less than the future: "The motivation of the desire to alienate and the desire for self-alienation is not only to make the proof of doubt and the conflict between the self and its ideals less insistent, less frequent or less dramatic. What those desires (or I would rather say that passion) intend is the sign of its excessiveness; that is, the exclusion of all causes of doubt, all causes of conflict and all causes of suffering" (p.19).

For Aulagnier (1993), one of the causes of this alienation turned into passion refers to the price that the self pays for renouncing the acceptance of reality and impossibility. An overly narcissistic self emerges on the basis of which there will be a 'prosthesis', which is the assessment of oneself and one's thoughts by another one that, in this case, is represented by medical technology and doctors, whose powers are massively idealized.

In short, alienation and passion as a drive destiny, from this perspective, allows us to understand the processes that exceed the desire for a child. They exceed showing a mixture of pleasure and suffering, of enjoyment also in the ART processes and pregnancy. Indeed, sometimes women insist on treatments, regardless of the collateral damage and the physical and emotional pain entailed.

The illness of ideality, a concept introduced by Chasseguet-Smirgel (2003), refers to the fixation in a longing for an ideal of happiness, which can turn into sublime achievements or madness. The parenting project may result in a necessity that would occupy that place-fixation of ideality. The super-ego, according to Freud's last model of mental functioning ([1926] 1994), is the place where ideals are found, carries out the command that becomes in "you must love the time of trying", as in Silvio Rodrigues's song.[2] Sometimes it will be a child; others, it will be the procedures; but what turns desire into passion? According to the author, it is the denial of the separation and the search for an erotic, aesthetic ideal. Particularly, it can be defined as the discovery of an object of devotion and self-sacrifice, like Geppetto's Pinocchio, or David's parents and his human brother.

The primary fusional illusion shows us the narcissistic imaginary origin. Thus, pregnancy and the baby become carriers of narcissistic satisfactions that bridge the gaps between the self of some women and their ideal: the way they would like to be. It is also observed the tyrannical deployment of cultural ideal imperatives that they assume as their own. It is as if we were returning to the lost narcissism of times of helplessness, in which pregnancy and the child represented a "promise of happiness".

This comes hand in hand with the freedom and rights conquered by women, like choosing when to be mothers and not necessarily following what cultural imperatives on family and motherhood establish. Frequently, when time does not expire and eggs can be kept frozen, we observe the transformation of desire into passion, the struggle of what Recalcati (2018) calls the *sentiment of life*; that is, the desire that tries not to succumb to passion. This author will use the term *Merversion*, and I think it is similar to what Patricia Alkolombre (2008) conceptualizes as passion; that desire for becoming and/or conceiving a child at all costs, which would not express a love-project-child, but rather something of the perverse order, which denies what is yearned. The son or daughter, during pregnancy and sometimes after being born, acts as an obturator for any lack and transcendence. He/she represents the closure of a monad whose existence depends on the maternal imaginary and on the reformulation, achievement or failure of the identification project of the woman-mother.

Final considerations

Recently, psychoanalysis has been studying the implications of technology in people's lives and in the analytical process. Since technology has developed from extending life to creating it, we still find ourselves travelling through unexplored territories. We are witnessing the confrontation of patients and analysts, as well as of the society as a whole, with complex human dilemmas for which, in many countries, there is not even legislation.

The passion for a child takes us to cyclical times of monotonous repetition: monitored ovulatory cycles, obsessive following of procedures, permeated with moments of doubt and anxiety. Moments experienced mainly by women, full of anguishing efforts to continue and succeed in the struggle against the difficulties and falls that characterize ART processes.

In our clinical work, in which we highlight and protect the uniqueness of each person and her experiences, we accompany patients who experience the passion for a child, and this in turn leads us to experience difficult medical, ethical and moral issues (Zalusky, 2000). Our own anxieties and fantasies are activated while we have to listen and help our patients to analyze theirs.

All the cited authors seem to agree that the intense stress of infertility may cause regressions to earlier stages of psychological development. We call them narcissistic, leaving the door open to primary envy, and subsequently, to psychic conflicts with roots found in childhood. The frightening feelings and fantasies that characterize fertilization attempts, resonating in nodal points of our psyche, can lead to the passion for a child.

In our work, from a transference perspective, we will try to turn the situation around or reach the other side of the Moebius strip, turning passion into desire, into love that recognizes reality and the other.

Many times, human beings will feel intense anxiety that doesn't allow them to think, and sometimes this leads to action. Maybe that's what our patients do; taking time in psychoanalysis to register emotions and understand anxieties allows the understanding of possible causes – creating narratives – which in turn provide enough calm to continue working for a desire and not for a passion.

Our work as psychoanalysts requires us to exercise patience; it isn't always sweet, of course sometimes it is very difficult and painful, but certainly it is libidinized and involves efforts to depathologize our listening. We must be always prepared for the unexpected to happen, so that we can contribute to the understanding of our patients, helping them to generate the necessary changes in their lives, and in ours of course.

Notes

1 *"Pasión de Hijo"* as it was originally coined in Spanish.
2 Reference to a Silvio Rodriguez's song "Debes amar" (you must love), a Cuban musician born in 1946 that was part of the movement Nova Trova Cubana.

References

Alkolombre, P. (2008). *Deseo de hijo. Pasión de hijo. Esterilidad y técnicas reproductivas a la luz del psicoanálisis.* Letra Viva.

Alkolombre, P. (2020). *Diccionario de psicoanálisis argentino. Nuevos términos. Volumen III* (pp. 355–357). Editorial de la Asociación Psicoanalítica Argentina.

Aulagnier, P. (1993). *Los destinos del placer. Alienación, amor, pasión.* Paidós.

Chasseguet-Smirgel, J. (2003). *El ideal del yo. Ensayo psicoanalítico sobre la "enfermedad de la idealidad".* Amorrortu.

Freud, S. ([1926] 1994). Inhibitions, symptoms and anxiety. In J. Strachey & A. Freud (Eds.), *The standard edition of the complete psychological works of Sigmund Freud, volume XX* (pp. 77–175). Hogarth Press.

Greil, A. L., Leitko, T. A., & Porter, K. L. (1988). Infertility: His and hers. *Gender & Society*, 2 (2): 172 – 199.

Klein, M. ([1935] 1998). A contribution to the psychogenesis of manic-depressive states. In *Love, guilt and reparation and other works* (pp. 262–289). Vintage.

Recalcati, M. (2018). *Las manos de la madre.* Anagrama.

Zalusky, S. (2000). Infertility in the age of technology. *Journal of the American Psychoanalytic Association*, 48 (4): 1541–1562.

Chapter 6

Emotional aspects of donors

Nancy Tame Ayub

The reproductive medicine field encompasses more than infertile patients seeking treatment. Many people are involved in it, such as doctors, nurses, family members, friends, psychoanalysts, psychotherapists and, particularly, donors.

The decision some women and men make to become donors is significant and deeply personal. Their participation in this reproductive medicine procedure and the ensuing emotional process they live can impact them in many ways. Undoubtedly, each decision and each story are unique.

This work is intended to reflect on that decision and on the emotional complexity of the procedure, which transcends a mere financial transaction and an economic agreement with the infertility clinic. In some cases, donors who took part in the procedure can go on with their life with no meaningful conflict; in other cases, years or decades after their experience at the infertility clinic, they may face a crisis that, in some cases, will have a profound impact on their lives.

Infertility affects 10–15% of couples and it is one of the most common conditions in 25–45-year-old individuals. The longer a woman tries to become pregnant without success, the less will her odds be of conceiving without initiating adequate treatment (ASRM, 2020).

Facing difficulty in having children can cause significant psychological pain, as well as physical burnout and financial downturn. From an economic perspective, treatments are expensive. Although some donors act for altruistic reasons, most of them get paid for their participation. Laws on the matter also vary. For example, in France, the 1994 law on bioethics ruled that donors had to already be parents; however, after being amended in 2011, it now allows that more men and women donate their gametes and candidates with no children are accepted (Bujan et al., 2022).

On the other hand, for those who decide to donate, this may mean taking a step into an unexplored territory in both psychological and physical terms (Fine, 2018).

The journey has been long. One of the earliest reported procedures of this kind is artificial insemination (AI), which has been practiced for centuries in order to reach a successful pregnancy. The procedure consists in depositing sperm into the uterus or the cervix by mechanical means.

DOI: 10.4324/9781032693446-6

Lazzaro Spallanzani, an Italian priest and physiologist (1729–1799), studied man's contribution to procreation. When experimenting with amphibians, he concluded that, for a new animal to develop, it is essential that sperm come into contact with the ovum. Spallanzani was a pioneer in studying and conducting experiments on what is now called AI, so he is considered its creator (Bozzini et al., 2016).

According to Spallanzani:

> The technique is very simple. It is just a matter of injecting the sperm into the vagina. Contrary to what most people think, you don't have to work with special light, air or heat conditions […] I have heard of a group of lesbian women […] who inseminated themselves using a kitchen tool, a syringe to inject the turkey […] I thought it was a great idea.
>
> (Wickler & Wickler, 1991, p.5)

Early critics of AI claimed that the practice was a sin, even if it was performed by a physician. In 1883, in France, a judge stated: "It is important for the dignity of marriage that these procedures not be transferred from the scientific field to the field of practice". Over time, as it became the responsibility of physicians – specifically those specialized in the subject – the insistence on the sinful aspect of this procedure subsided (Wickler & Wickler, 1991).

Upon qualifying as a medical procedure, artificial insemination was accepted and the perception of patients, professionals and society in this regard changed (Menning, 1988).

In Alkolombre and Holovko's terms:

> We can affirm that motherhood and fatherhood are no longer what they were and this is a process that cannot be reversed… *a new order of sexuality and reproduction* is built into the culture, new forms of interaction between genders are simultaneously enabled and power relations between men and women change.
>
> (2016, p. 65)

In 1884, in Philadelphia, doctor William Pancoast decided to conduct an experiment with a woman whose husband was infertile. He anesthetized her and, without requesting prior authorization from the couple, he inseminated her with sperm donated by a medical student he considered suitable and attractive (Mundy, 2008).

This seems to be the first case of AI with a donor's sperm. Although Pancoast informed her husband of the procedure, the patient never found out and died thinking that he was the biological father of her child. That experiment marked the beginning of the procedure that for many years was the only option available to overcome male infertility.

By 1900, in the United States and England, donor insemination had become a well-established practice. After World War II, many soldiers returned home with physical injuries, an issue that was sorted out using this increasingly common method. While physicians themselves could be the donors, good-looking medical students were usually asked to donate sperm. In some cases, the donor's sperm was mixed with that of the infertile father, a ritual that fueled the fiction that he might in fact be the biological father. About 30,000 children were born as a result of the procedure (Mundy, 2008).

Sperm freezing and thawing procedures were devised in the 1940s and started to be used in AI in 1950. The first pregnancy using frozen sperm was reported in 1953 (Kably et al., 2012). In the United States, most women under 40 years of age use their own eggs for this kind of insemination, while 73% of women 44 years of age and older choose to use donor eggs (Jensen & Stewart, 2015).

Some couples, as well as single women and men who decide to use assisted reproductive techniques, let their children know that they were conceived by donation, while others never do. Many parents do not explain this for fear of weakening the bond between them and of generating a strong internal conflict, or in an attempt to prevent the biological father from feeling "closer" and with more authority towards his offspring (Jaffe, Ourieff Diamond & Diamond, 2005). The guiding principle when selecting donors is critically important, as this type of programmed selection reveals and takes into account the wishes and fantasies of the prospective parents (Alizade, 2006).

During those months and years devoted to undergo infertility treatments, patients will have to make several decisions – very complex decisions in some cases – that will challenge their value system and bring out the expectations they had when their journey in search of parenthood started. Procedures that involve the participation of donors are ideal for some of these infertile patients, or for those who turn to infertility clinics without necessarily having reproductive issues – for example, single women and men or same-gender couples who aspire to become parents.

Infertile couples and those who choose the donation technique may live out fantasies before conception, during pregnancy and after their child is born. They may feel envy or gratitude towards the male or female donor, or a profound uncertainty about his/her identity and genetic load. They will probably not talk about the procedure they are going through and, before their relatives and friends, the pregnancy may seem the same as other couples' pregnancies; however, the presence of the male or female donor may linger in their mind for a long time. In some cases, partners have conflicts with each other because, after all, one of them is biologically related to their child while the other is not (Tame, 2016).

As pregnancy moves forward, doubts can escalate: "What if our decision was wrong? For example, how will the fact that the baby's ethnic group – or his/

her physical appearance – is different from ours affect us?" Donor infertility treatments open the door to a whole world of fantasies, fears and suspicion. What began as an opportunity offered by the medicine field's new findings and developments, can be experienced as the entrance to an unknown world in which the decision has already been made and there is no turning back (Tame, 2016).

Much has been done and researched aiming to alleviate the pain that many couples who, for one reason or another, are unable to have a child, endure. Based on these efforts, several alternatives emerged: a) adoption or surrogate motherhood, or b) clinical procedures, such as intrauterine insemination, sperm donation, in vitro fertilization (IVF) and egg or embryo donation.

Regarding the preceding, a case in point is that of a couple who for several years faced serious hardships to conceive a child, which triggered a painful feeling of loss. For a long time, they explored and reflected on the pros and cons of the different alternatives available. Finally, they decided to initiate infertility treatments and ended up participating in an egg donation program.

Egg donation made the desired pregnancy, and its positive completion, possible. However, later on, they started a psychoanalytic psychotherapy for couples, where they expressed that before and during the procedure, they did not even stop to thoroughly reflect on other matters related with the procedure in question. Within this context, they realized that their psychic energy, their efforts and their attention focused on the treatment and on being able to conceive. Meanwhile, surprisingly, the fear of having a child completely different from them increased and shifted to persecutory fantasies. For instance, although they had "chosen" a donor who shared similar characteristics, they wondered about their extended family's reactions: "Will they accept our child?", "Will their attitude towards us change?", "Will they judge us if they find out about the procedure undertaken?".

During the procedure they focused on their rational side, probably as a defense mechanism that would enable them to feel in control of the situation and maybe also to act driven by the illusion of "controlling" their emotions. However, what was really surprising was the intensity of the emotional reaction they faced later on.

In a psychoanalytical context, these anxiety episodes are not necessarily considered as related only to the actual situation. In fact, something else is being projected and other instances of the couple's history are linked to what they now experience. Psychoanalysis has shown that past and present times are intertwined and that the psychic system is dynamic. The egg donation process and the time waited during pregnancy, as well as the financial and the emotional burnout arising from so many years of treatment, combined to trigger a crisis driven by the donation's impact, but also by their fears and the fantasies they created related to their lives' story and their relationship as a couple.

Regarding the preceding, Michel Tort stated the following:

> The risk parents and children face as far as revealing the child's origin to others is concerned, is not the same as in adoption situations, since artificial insemination with donor indicates [...] the inequality in the biological "filiation" of the couple's child.
> But the issue raised by donor artificial insemination is not reduced to a practice enlightened by science and disconnected from the representation of inheritance. Basically, apart from scientific knowledge, it does what lies at the heart of filiation stories: the fabrication of a secret.
>
> (1992 p. 214)

The psychoanalytical proposal is the way the subject will position himself/herself in the face of his/her condition; the way this will be linked to his/her history; what sort of impact can this experience have throughout his/her life and how all these aspects will come into play in the transference and in the relationship that will be built with the psychoanalyst.

Some of the parties involved in a child's birth are visible, while others, such as donors, may remain anonymous. However, this certainly does not mean that their representation and their psychic impact do not exist and that they do not affect the future family. During and after the pregnancy, unconscious fantasies will be projected onto the female or male donor.

Who is the donor and what are his/her motivations?

Baran and Pannor, who conducted one of the first investigations on the psychological implications faced by young men that collaborated in donor insemination, reported the following case:

> A patient that consulted Dr. Phil told him he and his wife were having trouble conceiving a child; the problem was his and the option they were offered was donor insemination. Their infertility-specialized physician, with previous experience on the procedure, assured them that no one would have to know about the procedure, that it would be their secret, that their feelings toward their child would be the same as those for a child born without the help of a donor. The donor candidates chosen at his clinic were usually medical students, whose physical and intellectual conditions were thoroughly evaluated. "Phil kept silent during the consultation; he was well acquainted with the subject of donor insemination because he himself had been one of those subjects evaluated and approved by the infertility clinic".
>
> (1993, pp. 88–89)

After the consultation, he remembered his college years as a medical student and the fact that he had been one of the most successful donors in his group. A friend had once told him:

They specify the rules on a sheet of paper. You make fifty dollars a week for a few minutes of work, although, actually, it is not precisely work.

The clinic is looking for new donors and you fit in very well. They want average young people, not too tall, not too dark, not too light, not too big, not too small.

(Baran & Pannor, 1993, p. 89)

Although Phil was not comfortable with the proposal, after reflecting on the matter, he felt more inclined to accept it and collaborate with the clinic; after all, he needed the money. He was not able to figure out how he felt about it: perhaps he was embarrassed … or did he feel he was a very special person and didn't want anyone else to have this honor? He decided not to keep it a secret and talked about it openly with his friends and later on with his partners. "Being a donor was an acceptable occupation and, moreover, a way to help others" (Baran & Pannor, 1993, p. 91).

Upon his first attempt, the infertility clinic director informed him that he had struck gold: the woman was already pregnant and both she and her husband were very happy. Without thinking much about it, he just kept donating; it was like any other job. The issue came to mind occasionally and he considered it coolly, with no emotional load. "Being a donor became a routine process for Phil, who participated in it along several years, twice a week on average" (Baran & Pannor, 1993, p. 92). A way of avoiding the emotional impact is to rationalize the body as if it were a machine (Alizade, 2006).

The donor's motifs, which have been a matter for research and of great interest for society as a whole, can relate to representations of internal processes. Also, the ambivalence they felt at the beginning may turn around and change over time (Gilman, 2022).

During his senior year in college, Phil visited his parents, who asked him about his financial status, since he never requested their economic support. This immediately opened up the donation subject. His parents' silence surprised him; they did not openly express their disapproval, but it was obvious they did not enjoy finding out about his participation in such procedures. Later that night, his mother told him: "What you are selling is not only your sperm; these are our grandchildren and I will never get to see them or know who they are". "Phil felt as if something had hit him and unthought thoughts began coming up in his mind" (Baran & Pannor, 1993, p. 94).

The intense anguish he felt amazed him. "This was a symptom, but a symptom of what? It is the symptom what prevails as the agent […] it is the unconscious in full exercise" (Rocha, 2022, p. 4).

This concept may be relevant in Phil's case; after 25 years, he now reflects on those children living somewhere and understands this issue is harder for him every day. What kind of person would have made those donations without considering the issue from a more responsible perspective? What kind of *macho* was he, feeling so satisfied when told that his sample had been the best among his group? How many children had been born as a result of his donations? Phil admitted that it was quite likely that more than a dozen children of his lived in his community. He called the infertility clinics involved and confirmed that confidentiality was still an essential requirement in this procedure, although in some cases those involved may be interested and curious about finding him and getting to know him. "The idea that someday his children would decide to get married worried him; of course, he would have to check the birth background of the future spouses of his children" (Baran & Pannor, 1993, p. 95).

Fine (2018) explained that families may perceive that it is possible to control the issue of distance by keeping at bay the donor as an actual human being. In 2005, in Great Britain, this stance was modified and the anonymity requirement was removed. This change opened another possibility of identifying them and the half-siblings conceived and, as a consequence, the possibility that "the child born of these procedures invites those biologically-related strangers to become part of his/her life" (p. 114).

Also, some infertility clinics encourage donors to think that their participation in these procedures is part of a business deal and, therefore, his motives are economic in nature. Authors have stated that, as time went by and donors kept on collaborating with the clinic, "the donor's narrative was transformed and they now expressed an altruistic motivation" (Gilman, 2022, p. 229).

Another factor worth considering is that, according to the literature on the subject, the fact that gametes for donation and for reproductive purposes are available does not mean that the donors authorized their use for research purposes (Baía et al., 2019). The work and efforts dedicated for so many years in order to take also into account the donors' rights have implied following a long and challenging path.

One of the infertility clinics Phil contacted reported that they were conducting a research project on the emotional aspects of donors. When he realized that they would have the opportunity to talk about this experience and their feelings towards it, he decided to participate, and felt relieved almost immediately. "Typical donors tend to be single, still teenagers from an emotional point of view, and generally uncapable of understanding the emotional impact of being a donor nor the feelings reproduction implies, and that will come up years later" (Baran & Pannor, 1993, p. 96).

Psychoanalytic and psychotherapeutic work transcend verbal expression and can reach deeper levels of the mind and body, especially when facing experiences that could – in cases like this – surprise and bewilder people later on. According to Rocha (2022), "in psychoanalysis, the interpersonal relationship is simple: one person talks and the other one listens. And, as it turns out, talking will have an impact on their mind, but also on their body" (p. 6).

On the other hand, the children of single mothers who underwent a donation procedure, as well as the children of same-gender couples, might be more open and interested in finding out about their genetic origin. Families of this kind were somehow the first to talk more openly about donors and, in some cases, to get to know them. Also, heterosexual couples are increasingly willing to let their children know how they were conceived (Ludden, 2011, in Mann, 2014).

For years, attention focused mostly on the medical and scientific aspects of infertility. It is still assumed that when these treatments end, either on the patient's initiative or due to the doctor's recommendation, everything will be over. Psychoanalysis shows that such thinking might be a mistake. Memories and experiences come back, challenge people and are connected with other moments in their lives.

Rosen and Rosen (2005) reported that in most of the cases analyzed, donors – men and women – receive no information on who will receive their gametes. This scenario is very different from the adoption scenario, in which information between the parties is increasingly accessible (for example, in an open adoption). It is worth questioning if this means not thinking about the responsibility of taking care of donors. Apparently, post-donation effects are not sufficiently identified and monitored, and such lack of research and follow-up may be due to the secrecy which usually surrounds the decision and the procedure to be followed. Rosen and Rosen (2005, p. 94) questioned: "Is it better to keep the female or male donor in the dark?"

There are many perspectives from which to address this matter and one of them is reflecting on the concept of memory posed by Sigmund Freud. This is considered one of the core contributions of psychoanalysis, since it gives this notion another dimension, another level of profoundness and complexity that transcends cognitive memory, which involves the inner world, the transcription, the drive, the inner time, the body, the transference and the person's history.

In his *Letter 52* to his friend Wilhelm Fliess, Freud explained the following

> You know that I work under the assumption that our psychic mechanism was generated by successive layering, because from time to time the pre-existing material undergoes a *reordering* according to new linkages, a *retranscription* (*Unmischrift*). What is essentially new in my theory, that is, the theory that memory does not pre-exist in a simple manner, but in a multiple manner, is captured in several kinds of signs.
>
> ([1896] 1988, p. 274)

The psychic apparatus is dynamic, it is not stationary. In this work, Freud talked to Fliess of a core aspect in the life of a human being: re-signification.

An action that at one stage in their lives was merely a business deal gets to be re-signified later on in an absolutely different manner, when considering the decision of becoming a donor with greater awareness and connecting such decision with affect at another level of intensity. At some point in their life, male and female donors, and each person involved in these procedures – including those psychoanalysts and psychotherapists they work with – may face their participation in them and the way in which they perceive them, feel them, interpret them and connect them with their story.

Another example is that of a nurse who worked in an infertility clinic and who had been an egg donor while in college, before getting married and having children. When interacting with many couples receiving donations, she admitted she had been unprepared for the types of behavior she would encounter in some patients and worried about what had happened with her eggs, who received them and where had they ended up. "This is a perspective few donors have, but it does point to an important party whose interests might be considered … along with those of the recipient couples and the potential children" (Rosen & Rosen, 2005, p. 94). Later on, when she had her own children, these thoughts grew stronger and her anxiety about the issue increased (Rosen & Rosen, 2005).

Psychoanalysis is a very helpful tool to understand the emotional aspect of a man or a woman who decides to become a donor, as well as to face the emotional reactions that may arise years after this experience took place. Indeed, some female and male donors may regard donation as a financial transaction, as an altruistic act or as an arrangement with the clinic, and, consequently, this event may not be the cause of conflict, at least not consciously. But in other cases, the reaction may be intense and complex. Therefore, it is necessary to explore the emotional process lived by male and female participants in infertility clinics' donation programs.

In conclusion, it is worth reflecting on the desire of a person to have children and on what occurs when an infertility problem comes up, that is, when the body does not adequately perform one of its functions specifically related to femininity and masculinity. As psychoanalysis has pointed out, the inner world has another pace and another kind of movement, it does not move forward at the same fast pace of science. Therefore, male and female donors may live very difficult times if thoughts, feelings, memories and emotional responses that they never imagined would linger in their mind arise.

At the beginning of this chapter, we stated that the decision to become a male or female donor is significant and deeply personal. Exploring the complexity of the inner world, the notion of memory, the internal time – other than chronological time – as well as questioning if emotions and emotional responses can really control a situation and the way experiences can be re-signified throughout our life has been one of the great contributions of psychoanalysis. The emotional impact caused by the clinical procedures we have addressed can be profound and complex and can amaze not only patients, but also other people who, one way or the other, get involved in the world of infertility.

References

Alizade, M. (2006). *Motherhood in the Twenty-First Century*. Karnac.
Alkolombre, P. & Holovko, C. (2016). *Parentalidades y género*. Letras Libres.
American Society for Reproductive Medicine (ASRM). (2020). Available online in www.asmr.org

Baía, I., De Freitas, C., Samorinha, C., Provoost, V. & Silva, S. (2019). Dual Consent? Donors' and recipients' views about involvement in decision making on the use of embryos created by gamete donation in research. *BMC Medical Ethics*, 20(90). https://doi.org/10.1186/s12910-019-04306

Baran, A. & Pannor, R. (1993). *Lethal secrets. The psychology of donor insemination.* Amistad.

Bozzini, G., Seveso, M., Bono, P., De Francesco, O., Mandressi, A., Taverna, G. y Castellanza, VA. (2016). History of urology: History forum II. *The Journal of Urology*, 195(4S), Suplemento 8 de mayo.

Bujan, L., Nouri, N., Papaxanthos-Roche, A., Ducrocq, B., Brugnon, F., Ravel, C., Rives, N., Teletin, M., Drouineaud, V., Delepine, B., Berthaut, I., Meltzer-Guillemain, C., Devaux, A., Frapsauce, C., Thibault, E., Blagosklonov, O., Clarotti, MA, Diligent, C., Loup Cabaniols, V.,... & Daudin, M. (2022). Motivations and personality characteristics of candidate sperm and oocyte donors according to parenthood status: A national study from the French CECOS network. *Human Reproduction Open*, 1–14.

Fine, K. (2018). *Donor conception for life.* Routledge.

Freud, S. ([1896] 1988). Fragmentos de la correspondencia con Fliess. In *Obras Completas. Tomo I.* (p. 274). Amorrortu.

Gilman, L. (2022). The "selfish element" - How sperm and egg donors construct plausibly moral accounts of the decision to donate. *Sociology*, 56(2): 227–243. DOI 10.1177/00380385211033153

Jaffe, J., Ourieff Diamond, M. & Diamond, D. (2005). *Unsung lullabies.* St. Martin Griffin.

Jensen, J. & Stewart, E. (2015). Mayo Clinic. In *Guide to Fertility and Conception.* Mayo Foundation for Medical Research (MFMER).

Kably Ambe, A., Salazar López, C., Serviere Zaragoza, C., Velázquez Cornejo, G., Pérez Peña, E., Santos Haliscack, R., Luna Rojas, M., Valerio, E., Santana, H. & Gaviño Gaviño, F. (2012). Consenso Nacional Mexicano de Reproducción Asistida. *Revista Mexicana de Medicina de la Reproducción*, 5(2): 68–113.

Mann, M. (2014). *Psychoanalytic aspects of assisted reproductive technology.* Routledge.

Menning, B. (1988). *Infertility. A guide for the childless couple.* Prentice Hall Press.

Mundy, L. (2008). *Everything conceivable.* Anchor Books.

Rocha, S. (2022). Hacia una genealogía del psicoanálisis (en México). *Psicología, educación & sociedad*, 1(1): 1–8. Available online https://revistas.uaq.mx/index.php/psicologia/article/view/851/758

Rosen, A. & Rosen, J. (2005). *Frozen dreams.* The Analytic Press.

Tame, N. (2016). *Infertilidad.* Grijalbo.

Tort, M. (1992). *El deseo frío.* Nueva Visión.

Wickler, D. & Wickler, N. J. (1991). Turkey baster babies: The demedicalization of artificial insemination. *The Milbank Quarterly*, 69(1): 5–44.

Chapter 7

Live babies and dead babies
Pregnancy and pregnancy loss in analysis

Ana Teresa Vale

Pregnancy as transformation

Pregnancy is a big event in a woman's life, both internally and externally, that demands change and transformation. From the moment a woman starts trying to get pregnant until the end of breast feeding, this is an emotionally intense period that brings to the fore unconscious fantasies and conflicts that were often inaccessible before, fostering a regression in all areas of mental functioning. Each woman's unique constellation of intrapsychic conflicts, emotions and fantasies will determine the nature and intensity of the emotional experience of pregnancy (Leon, 1990).

In the midst of this turmoil, which implies a recapitulation of the infantile sexuality, there are several aspects of the woman's psyche that suffer a profound change – her identity, her relationship to her body, her relationship to the maternal object, her narcissistic equilibrium, just to name a few. All this psychic work often leads to a mental reorganization of the woman's inner world (Deutsch, 1945; Pines, 1972, 1990; Leon, 1990; Raphael-Leff, 2015; Barandiaran, 2022).

In analysis, when the analyst has the privilege to witness this work of transformation, the transference and countertransference relationship also changes and is very often a situation of intense growth for both parties.

All pregnancies comprise a degree of anxiety, connected to unconscious and conscious fears of different types – one of the most common being the fear of the baby's death. Every pregnancy, being the source of a new life, is at the same time the battleground between life and death. For this reason, the idea of death is always present when a woman is pregnant, in different degrees and assuming different forms according to the woman's personality and past experiences.

This phenomenon can be read on the oedipal level – getting pregnant rises the woman to the level of the mother, which in the unconscious mind always contains some degree of danger.

Therefore, the oedipal rivalry is present, together with the guilt feelings that it entails, and in the unconscious fantasy the baby's death could be the punishment to be expected (Shulman, 2018).

DOI: 10.4324/9781032693446-7

On a pre-oedipal level, the fantasy of the baby's death is connected to the representation of the archaic mother, who has the power over life and death. On one hand, the pregnant woman fears the archaic mother inside her and the potential destructivity this figure represents; on the other hand, the pregnant woman, becoming a mother, also identifies with the maternal object, leading to unconscious fears of her own destructivity. The baby's death could in the unconscious fantasy be the result of this destructivity (Reenkola, 2022; Vale, 2020, 2022).

Finally, this fear of the baby's death can also come from an unconscious death wish. It is important to point out that a degree of hatred always is present in any mother towards any child, as Winnicott (1949) reminds us, because in some degree the baby is seen as threatening for the mother – a threat to her life and to her body, a threat to her physical as well as psychical well-being, a threat to life as she knew it and that no longer is. Moreover, when she has had a painful relationship with her maternal figure, the woman may fear she will repeat what she has experienced with her mother as a child (Shulman, 2018).

At the same time, pregnancy and the continuation of one's heritage is also a way to avoid death and brings a feeling of something that will endure after the parents are gone. In that sense, giving life is also felt as a way to defeat death (Deutsch, 1945; Leon, 1990). So we can see that in the creation of a new life the idea of death is present at different levels and with different meanings.

Pregnancy loss and the fear of the baby's death

All these unconscious movements can be subtle, only emerging through the fleeting fear that something is wrong with the baby in the womb or that something will go wrong while giving birth. Or they can be very intense, transforming the experience of being pregnant into something very painful and sometimes terrifying.

This is more often the case when the woman is pregnant after having suffered a pregnancy loss. In these cases, the fantasy of the baby's death becomes a reality and, as we know from investigation and literature, in the pregnancy that follows anxiety will be particularly present and intense, amplifying fears, emotions and fantasies that are already a part of any pregnancy (Leon, 1990; Squires, 2002; Quagliata, 2008, 2013; Alvarez, Yamgnane, Disnan, & Squires, 2009; Nayar-Akhtar, 2018).

The pregnancy loss can then be felt as a punishment for illicit oedipal desires or as a confirmation that there is an internal mother that attacks the woman's resources and competences, forbidding her to become a mother. In fact, the impact of pregnancy loss is profound and lasting, leading to very difficult emotions to cope with – shock, pain, anger, emptiness, despair, loneliness, guilt, helplessness, worthlessness (Leon, 1990; Squires, 2002; Quagliata, 2013, Raphael-Leff, 2015; Nayar-Akhtar, 2018; Shulz & Soubieux, 2018; Barandiaran, 2022; Vale, 2022; Vives, 2022).

As Leon (1996a) points out, the pregnancy loss is both the loss of a loved one and the loss of a dream. Like other losses, the pregnancy loss brings to the fore past experiences of loss and mourning, but in this specific case, the lost loved one has no face, no identity. Therefore, often the dead baby represents a dead or agonizing part of the mother's self (as conceptualized by Ferenczi 1995), especially when the loss activates other infantile trauma.

For that reason, his/her representation in the mother's mind gets mixed up with that of other people in one's life that one has lost. This led Deutsch (1945) and other authors after her (Aguiar & Zornig, 2016) to postulate that the pregnancy loss was not an actual loss, but mainly the loss of a fantasy. On the contrary, what we see in our clinical practice, corroborated by other authors (Leon, 1990, 1996a; Quagliata, 2013; Vives, 2022), is that often the woman that suffers a pregnancy loss represents what she has lost as a baby (despite the gestational age of the child). Moreover, most women give him/her an object status and mourn their loss as such, and therefore this loss is not felt as just the loss of a fantasy or project.

Quagliata (2008) clearly describes the traumatic experience of recurrent pregnancy loss, which brings to the fore identity fragilities, which the author seems to locate at the level of psychic separation from the maternal object. This fragility makes the woman feel worthless, depleted of any creative capability (which further weakens identity).

The author also highlights the presence of an internal enemy, a deadly internal object that forbids the subject to grow up, to become a woman and a mother. The woman feels hopeless and lonely, with no trust in her ability to generate a live baby inside her, as if crushed by an inexorable destiny. Moreover, the identification to the dead baby (in order not to lose him/her completely) can unleash a catastrophic anxiety, bringing to the fore the psychotic aspects of the personality (Squires, 2002).

The relationship between the mind and the body becomes disturbed. The body is felt as an enemy that betrays the woman by joining forces with the deadly internal object that does not allow her and her babies to grow. The patient feels she has lost control of her own body, picturing it as a place of death instead of life. Simultaneously, all the suffering and sorrow is registered in the body, and her reaction to these bodily manifestations depends on the meanings she attributes to her loss and her symptoms (Leon, 1990; Quagliata, 2008; Ramos & Canta, 2020; Vives, 2022).

According to the personality structure, these emotions will have different effects and incite different defense mechanisms, leading to several symptoms, more or less severe, including depression, anxiety, panic attacks, psychosomatic symptoms, sexual symptoms, amongst others (Ramos & Canta, 2020).

In a relationship as profound and complex as the analytic relationship, it is expected that all these emotions are received and felt by the analyst while she walks besides her patient, accompanying her mourning and suffering. As Squires (2002) points out, the elaboration of the counter-transferential movements is crucial; the anxiety and pain the analyst finds within herself is connected to the way she herself deals with death, loss, loneliness, failure and the way she tolerates what remains unexplained.

There are some situations where the fear of the baby's death is so intense that it attacks the analyst's mind, communicating by projective identification a very intense terror, not yet worked through. It will be the analyst's job to process the best she can these undigested emotions – these beta elements to use Bion's terminology (Symington & Symington, 1999) – and try to deliver to the patient an interpretation that can be useful, meaningful and not anxiety-inducing, keeping in mind that the patient is in a very delicate situation and mental state.

Lydia and the omnipotent destructive mother

Lydia came to analysis at a time of her life when she felt great anxiety about two situations – her difficult relationship with her family, namely her mother and siblings, and her difficult relationship to her small child, to whom she felt less available and tolerant than she would like to.

In our first meetings, Lydia talked about her destructive mother, always disgruntled. She also mentioned her very difficult obstetric history. When she first got pregnant, a malformation was diagnosed, and she had to decide to terminate her pregnancy. We know from the literature on the subject (Leon, 1990) that this kind of parental decision, when it is caused by an abnormal medical diagnostic, is emotionally felt like a pregnancy loss. In fact, this was a very difficult mourning for Lydia, and she could not get pregnant again for more than a year.

When she finally got pregnant again, the cervix revealed to be incompetent and started to give in too early, when she was just seven months pregnant. She was admitted to the hospital in high risk of premature labour, at a time when the baby was still not viable.

Threatened with the loss of her second baby, Lydia clung to the conviction that she would win this battle and hold her live baby in her arms against all odds. She stayed in the hospital for several weeks, and afterwards she went home, and was able to bring the pregnancy to term, and a healthy boy was born.

But then, astonished, she found the relationship with the baby to be very frustrating. Before she had a baby, she imagined that the first few months would be chaotic and later her controlled life would go back to normal. Of course, that is not what a baby brings to anyone's life. When she came to analysis, she was still very frustrated, angry and discouraged by the child's dependency on her.

As the analysis unfolded, we started to understand the helplessness and loneliness she had felt as a child, and her melancholic core, linked to a destructivity very difficult to grasp, that I first sensed through my countertransference. Whenever I made some interpretation concerning this issue, she would answer that she couldn't see what I was talking about.

Nonetheless, some internal changes happened in analysis and at this point, she got pregnant again, after two years of unsuccessful attempts. She was thrilled about the pregnancy. In the sessions, I tried to point out some ambivalence (fears related to pregnancy, or to what could come after, fear of having unfulfilled expectations) but she cut me short: "Probably what you point out is there, but when I think about this baby, the only thing I can think of is that he is here to make my family whole, to give me strength."

Some physical symptoms appeared in the first few weeks, and she was asked to stay at home resting by her doctor, so we went online. In this new setting, she kept rejecting all my attempts to explore the fantasies that could be connected to the baby growing inside her. I grew more and more aware of an uneasiness that was building up inside me, without being able to describe it properly. Only later, during an in-person session, I understood my emotion.

On that day, the patient arrived and lay on the couch, telling me she just came from the second trimester ultrasound. She mentioned the cervix had decreased from one week to the next, which made me feel alarmed and worried, but the doctor didn't think much of it. She went on describing several medical details and the uneasiness that I had been feeling grew inside me even more. I asked her if she had been resting as the doctor ordered, and she described the work she had been doing around the house and in the garden – and by then I was very alarmed.

At that moment, thinking that she was not considering the risks she was taking, suddenly I understood that I was filled with fear of death. The idea of the baby's death had been on my mind for some time and had finally emerged to consciousness.

When I tried to translate my feeling into words, she answered: "I am so convinced that this pregnancy will go well that I refuse to go into that mindset where I cannot do this, I cannot do that. I just want to have a normal pregnancy".

The patient's answer scared me a lot. I realized that I was experiencing the fear of death that the patient was at that point unable to feel, defended as she was by her omnipotent stance. To protect herself and the baby from the damage caused by her own destructivity, it was as if she had to resort to an omnipotent defense, in which she believed she was in control of everything. In her mind, at this point, there was no risk, no ambivalence.

From my perspective, this omnipotent defense was joining forces with the deadly mother inside her. I felt I had a dilemma to solve – should I make an interpretation highlighting this destructive part that I believed to be in action, in this very delicate moment, knowing that the patient did not want to hear about it? I decided not to, but the doubt lingered.

The session ended and I felt very worried and afraid, asking myself if I should not have told the patient what I thought was happening. After the session, Lydia suffered a pregnancy loss, followed by a serious hemorrhage that was only solved by an uterus excision. When I received the news, I felt a heavy weight on my chest, as if I was crushed by something very heavy.

When she returned to the sessions, that was precisely the feeling she described – betrayed, ran over, lost in the void of hopelessness. She was very angry and with scarce motivation to keep on living. She described the day of her admission to the hospital, and it was clear to both of us that a deadly force had been operating – she had understood that something was wrong, but she did not seek help. She felt that this fight against death (and against her destructivity) was out of her reach.

She related that feeling, and the choice she had made, with the destructive part of her personality that I had mentioned previously. But she was also very angry with the doctor, with the nurses, with the analyst – because analysis gave her hope she could fight the deadly forces inside her and win; but after all, the analyst was not an omnipotent mother that could guarantee her that victory.

The following sessions (that remain online) are very painful to us both and tears come to my eyes several times. I felt powerless, without knowing what could be said, or done, to help the patient in such a tragic moment, facing such a dramatic loss: not just the loss of that baby, but of any other future baby, and the loss of such an important part of her female body.

I decided to just listen, allowing her to voice her anger, her despair, her suffering, the profound narcissistic blow she was feeling, and the immense loneliness that nothing nor no one could mitigate.

She desperately needed me to hold her, but I tried to do it and could not get through to her. It was as if she was a premature baby in an incubator and I could not touch her. She responded to my interpretation by saying that was exactly what she never had – the cervix that could not hold the baby inside her was equivalent to her mother's arms that never held her. Lydia cried and showed me her profound suffering but at the same time she remained inaccessible, aloof.

Eventually, the patient decided she was not able to continue. She was not motivated to maintain the analysis because she at that point expected nothing from life. We were in a stalemate situation, that she solved by dropping out, leaving the analyst with a feeling of loss that seemed irredeemable. I felt frustrated and defeated.

Pregnancy loss has a huge impact on many levels that should be explored and clarified, but that cannot happen immediately after the tragic event. As Leon (1990) points out, in the period right after the loss, it is more useful to the grieving woman to be heard and understood, to have her emotions accepted unconditionally without judgment (even without what could be felt as judgment, as an explanatory interpretation – this loss happened because …).

The work of mourning must be done, at least partially, so that the more in-depth unconscious aspects can be explored. That was what Lydia could not do with me, because she unconsciously felt me as a destructive mother: one who first gave her hope, only to destroy it afterwards.

But I was also left with many questions unanswered: did my feeling of powerlessness put me in a position towards the patient where nothing could be done? Maybe my gentleness, avoiding interpreting certain aspects that I sensed were at stake, although they were threatening, was in fact my own defense against this profound anxiety and fear of death the patient brought to the field, which had a big resonance inside me. I felt that this was also my responsibility, as if I could have prevented this terrible loss.

Probably nothing could have prevented this pregnancy's dramatic outcome because a severe obstetric complication was diagnosed in the baby's autopsy. But the feeling that the analyst was left with was that she had not done all she could to guarantee this pregnancy's successful outcome.

Marina and the psychotic identification with the dead baby

Marina was in analysis for 5 years when she suffered three early-term pregnancy losses, following her first attempt to get pregnant. These miscarriages triggered several emotions and fantasies – on one hand, this meant to her that she was like her mother (who had lost a baby when she was a child), and so she needed to go through this pain of loss and death before she could give birth to a live baby. On the other hand, these events made her feel desperate, afraid and feeling less a woman than the rest of us (a feeling that she had always had, and thus in her mind the reality confirmed her fears).

Another aspect of her reaction to what was happening to her came up as a guilt feeling because she might have killed her babies (because she smoked or had taken drugs or sleeping pills in the past). For her that might mean that unconsciously she did not want a baby. This led us to understand that she had to come to terms with the image of a destructive mother that kills babies instead of nurturing them – and that made her feel terrified of her mother, of me in the transference and of herself, of the potential destructivity she felt in women in general, and in her analyst/mother in particular.

After the miscarriages followed a period of infertility – she couldn't get pregnant and the doctors that she reached out to couldn't tell her why. In analysis, she would ask me if her emotional conflicts were the cause of her infertility and had the fantasy that she couldn't get pregnant due to her destructivity, which entailed a great mental pain. As an analyst, I was left with the anxiety and sorrow of not having an answer to give her and not having the miraculous interpretation that could solve her problem. At this point, she trusted me to help her get through this difficult experience, but at the same time her suspicion towards her analyst was displaced to the medical doctors and obstetricians that couldn't find why she wouldn't get pregnant.

In the beginning of 2020, she finally got pregnant again. At first she was happy but very soon she started to worry – we were already getting news about the coronavirus in China and she immediately built up the fantasy that she would get the virus and it would kill her baby.

With the lockdown, the sessions went online. She was in a mental state that I had never seen in her before – in Klein's terms (1946), she had regressed to the paranoid-schizoid position and her thought process was very concrete, her dreams very poor and she was constantly invaded by the fear of the baby's death. It was very near to a psychotic delusion (a part of her "knew" the baby was going to die) but at the same time she still could understand that those were fantasies and not realities.

She craved our sessions more than ever, because during our sessions she could voice all her fantasies of her and the baby dying, she could talk about her terror and the intense pain she was feeling. Apart from the sessions, everyone else around her was terrified and exhausted by her constant insistence that she would get COVID and the baby would die, so she felt she had to conceal (at great cost and not very efficiently) what she was thinking and feeling. She then used the sessions to vomit all these horrible fantasies, all these undigested emotions, and the sessions were very difficult to me as an analyst. She was expecting me to convince her that her fantasies were not real, but nothing I said could reassure her.

Throughout the pregnancy, I was living with this dead baby inside my head, struggling to keep my patient and her baby emotionally alive. The sessions were filled with concrete details about COVID and COVID–related news and I saw in my patient no emotional bond to the baby, which worried me a lot and made me fear a post-partum depression. As several authors highlight (Quagliata, 2008; Alvarez et al., 2009), the investment in this pregnancy was clearly leaning more towards the dead babies than to the live one in her womb.

My countertransference oscillated between a fear of her and her baby's well-being (sometimes I feared she would not recover her emotional resources), an intense irritation because it was very hard to listen to the same ruminations over and over again, and a profound sadness for what she was going through. It was the most painful pregnancy I ever witnessed and this thought came to my mind several times: "No one should experience a pregnancy like this one".

Death was always around – the fear of the baby's death, which evoked the death of her sibling when she was a child; the fear that my patient wouldn't recover emotionally (which symbolically was like the Marina I knew had died); the death of the analytic relationship as we knew it, as the sessions unfolded in a repetitive, tiresome and frightening way, seemingly without any progress.

The baby was born prematurely and needed a few days in the incubator. After that, quickly I began to see an active, enthusiastic baby, who made his needs very clear. Nonetheless, the mother was not in a good shape emotionally. A part of her mind was still detached from her baby, but at the same time she was working hard to recover, to bond with her baby, to become the mother she feared she couldn't be. Again, as we had understood after the pregnancy losses, she was struggling with an internal mother that wouldn't allow her to grow up and become a mother.

But we also came to understand that this psychotic-like functioning she was showing during pregnancy and post-partum was simultaneously an identification to her and her mother's lost babies and a profound and hidden identification to her psychotic grandmother. In fact, the grandmother had been a present and important person in the patient's childhood, and she had witnessed the grandmother's psychic breakdown on more than one occasion. Although never properly diagnosed, these breakdowns were paranoid and delusional and had a profound impact on Marina.

Slowly she started to get out of that state. When the maternity leave was over, she resumed her professional life and started to get in touch more and more with reality, leaving the delusion-like thoughts behind. This opened the path to a more profound bond with her baby. But as she deepened her understanding about what had happened to her, she had to come to terms with the fact that the first few months of this relationship were very difficult and she was very far from the mother she wanted to be to her newborn child.

Pregnancy is a very delicate moment, which can be thought of as an overload both to the mind and to the body. As the body has to deal with so much more than when there is no pregnancy, also the mind has a lot more going on in terms of emotions, fantasies, fears. As other intense emotional experiences, this overload can lead to a psychic rupture, as was Marina's case, or mobilize psychic resources that will lead to transformation and growth.

In Marina's case, fortunately we were able to survive to this rupture and eventually work it through. Several questions linger still in my mind – if she hadn't experienced the pregnancy losses before the birth of her baby, would she have experienced the following pregnancy the same way? If we were not in the start of the pandemic, would she have had the same emotional reaction to pregnancy? We'll never know.

But I think the overload that caused a rupture and regression in her mind came from not just the pregnancy in itself, but also from the traumatic sequela of the pregnancy losses and the traumatic shock of the pandemic, which made her go back to the trauma of her childhood, mainly connected to her sibling's death and the consequences it brought to her family.

Marina's case makes us wonder whether the conflicts she had previously around femininity, motherhood and the relationship to her internal mother were an etiological factor on the pregnancy losses (such explanations are suggested by Deutsch, 1945; Pines, 1972, 1990; but are contradicted by authors as Leon, 1990, 1996b; Apfel & Keylor, 2002; Nayar-Akhtar, 2018). But the fact is that, despite all the intense ambivalence, terror, pain, during pregnancy, she was able to give birth to a healthy and competent baby.

I'm more inclined to think that the pregnancy losses activated and exacerbated conflicts and fragilities that she already had, and even after years of work, when she got pregnant, in the beginning of the pandemic, was too much for her mind to handle.

She regressed to a paranoid-schizoid functioning, making clear to the analyst something she had hinted before but had never understood completely – the identification with a psychotic grandmother. This aspect of her mind explained some symptoms she had experienced in childhood and adolescence that were finally clarified in depth.

From the analyst's side, it felt like a battle between life and death. I held in my mind the image of the Marina I knew from before and the emotional resources I knew she had, and I was constantly fighting against the dead parts inside her mind, that sometimes seemed strong enough to take her, her baby and the analysis down the drain. I was the depository of her sane and competent parts and my task was to make sure they didn't die. I can't affirm that it was the work of analysis that allowed this baby to be born; but I'm sure it was the work of analysis that allowed Marina to get out of her insane state of mind and finally bond with her baby.

Final considerations

Pregnancy is a very intense and complex period of a woman's life. Although usually associated with thrill, excitement, happiness, bliss, it also entails some degree of anxiety, fear, discomfort, sometimes even disgust and terror. In analysis, when a patient gets pregnant, it is usually felt by the analyst as an achievement and she shares with her patient these blissful, happy feelings.

But her experience as a woman and as an analyst also calls her attention to the dangers and difficulties a pregnancy may bring, to the analytic process and to the pregnant woman herself.

When the terror, anxiety and ideas of death are prevalent in the pregnant woman's mind and in the psychoanalytic field, this can be a very turbulent and painful period. It might turn into an obstacle to the analytic process, leading to unbearable experiences and eventually to drop outs.

In fact, the analyst's mind might be bombarded by the fear of the baby's death or by the representation of the dead baby (calling forth her own life and/or obstetric history), which is a mental content very difficult to hold on to. The working-through of these situations first starts in the mind of the analyst, before it can have an effect on the patient. In fact, when a pregnancy is this painful, the patient is not capable of thinking these thoughts or getting in touch with these fantasies, so it must be the analyst that keeps inside her mind these terrifying contents.

In that sense, it is also an opportunity to break through certain unconscious defenses, since it brings to consciousness something that was in most cases inaccessible before. This can lead to an exploration of very deep layers of the patient's mind, that may strengthen the patient's feminine identity, establish a better narcissistic equilibrium, and transform deeply her relationship to her maternal object, all allowing the patient to become a good-enough mother.

Surviving this assault to her mind, the analyst can also feel a good enough mother to her patient, nurturing the analytic process and allowing growth for both parties involved.

References

Aguiar, H. & Zornig, S. (2016). Luto fetal: A interrupção de uma promessa. *Estilos Clínicos*, 21: 264–281. https://doi.org/0.11606/issn.1981-1624.v21i2p264-281

Alvarez, L., Yamgnane, A., Disnan, G., Squires, C. (2009) Destins du deuil périnatal: Un cas clinique. *Champ Psychosomatique, L'esprit du temps, Destins de naissance*, 4: 53–70. https://doi.org/10.3917/cpsy.056.0053

Apfel, R. & Keylor, R. (2002). Psychoanalysis and infertility – Myths and realities. *International Journal of Psychoanalysis*, 83: 85–104. https://doi.org/10.1516/00207 57021601702

Barandiaran, S. (2022). El tabú de la maternidad. *Revista de Psicoanálisis de la Asociación Psicoanalítica de Madrid*, 97: 423–445.

Deutsch, H. (1945). *The psychology of women, volume 2 – Motherhood*. Grune & Stratton.

Ferenczi, S. (1995). *The clinical diary of Sandor Ferenczi*. Harvard University Press.

Leon, I. (1990). *When a baby dies – Psychotherapy for pregnancy and newborn loss*. Yale University Press.

Leon, I. (1996a). Revising psychoanalytic understanding of perinatal loss. *Psychoanalytic Psychology*, 13: 161–176. https://doi.org/10.1037/h0079646

Leon, I. (1996b). Reproductive loss: Barriers to psychoanalytic treatment. *Journal of the American Academy of Psychoanalysis*, 24: 341–352.

Klein, M. (1946) Notes on some schizoid mechanisms. *International Journal of Psychoanalysis*, 27: 99–110.

Nayar-Akhtar, M. (2018). Infertility, trauma and assisted reproductive technology: Psychoanalytic perspectives. In M. Mann (Ed.). *Psychoanalytic aspects of assisted reproductive technology* (pp. 77–95). Routledge.

Pines, D. (1972). Pregnancy and motherhood: Interaction between fantasy and reality. *British Journal of Medical Psychology*, 45: 333–343.

Pines, D. (1990). Pregnancy, miscarriage and abortion. A psychoanalytic perspective. *International Journal of Psychoanalysis*, 71: 301–313.

Quagliata, E. (2008). *A psychoanalytic study of recurrent miscarriage – Brief psychotherapeutic work with pregnant women*. Doctorate Thesis in Psychoanalytic Psychotherapy awarded by the University of East London in partnership with the Tavistock and Portman NHS Foundation Trust.

Quagliata, E. (2013). A paradoxical pain: Recurrent miscarriage. In E. Quagliata (Ed.), *Becoming parents and overcoming obstacles* (pp. 11–22). Karnac.

Raphael-Leff, J. (2015). *Dark side of the womb*. Grosvenor Group.

Ramos, V. & Canta, G. (2020). Perda e luto fetal. *Revista Portuguesa de Psicanálise*, 40: 29–35. https://doi.org/10.51356/rpp402a2

Reenkola, E. (2022). Envy between women. *The Scandinavian Psychoanalytic Review*, 44: 59–66. https://doi.org/10.1080/01062301.2022.2137312

Shulman, T. (2018). Psychoanalytic treatment of anxiety related to motherhood and the use of assisted reproductive technology. In M. Mann (Ed.). *Psychoanalytic aspects of assisted reproductive technology* (pp. 45–61). Routledge.

Shulz, J. & Soubieux, M. (2018). *Le deuil prénatal*. Féderation Wallonie-Bruxelles de Belgique.

Squires, C. (2002). Les psychothérapies périnatales lors d'une mort fœtale in utero: L'angoisse du clinicien face aux angoisses de mort. L'analyse du contre-transfert. In M. Bydlowski, C. Squires, D. Candilis (Eds.). *Des mères et leurs nouveau-nés. Recherche et interventions autour de la naissance*. Editions E.S.F.

Symington, N. & Symington, J. (1999). *O pensamento clínico de Wilfred Bion*. Climepsi.

Vale, A. (2020). A morte, a perda e o feminino – O impacto da perda gestacional da analista no processo psicanalítico. In R. Degani, S. Heissler, J. Lima, G. Seben & M. Camargo (Eds.). *A analista grávida* (pp. 99–115). Artes & Ecos.

Vale, A. (2022). A perda gestacional na análise – Aspetos contratransferenciais. In R. Vives (Ed.). *Ensaios sobre reprodução assistida, parentalidades e adoção – volume 2* (pp. 32–45). Génese Editora.

Vives, R. (2022). O corpo que sangra, o bebé que se vai – Dores da reprodução assistida. In XV Dialogo Cowap, July 2022, online conference titled "Mujer, género, cultura, futuro".

Winnicott, D. (1949). Hate in the counter-transference. *The International Journal of Psychoanalysis, 30*: 69–74.

Chapter 8

As good as it gets

Psychoanalysis as a fertile encounter

Conceição Tavares de Almeida

Introduction

Infertility is a complex and distressing reality for many individuals and couples worldwide. Beyond the physiological aspects, infertility often unravels rooted conflicts as well as imparts significant psychological effects. Through psychoanalysis, shedding light on the psychological dimension of infertility, it becomes possible not only to comprehend its impact, but also to explore the ways in which the whole process of working through during clinical approach can both highlight and repair those aspects. In this work we will look at clinical material to identify singular personal stories, theoretical frameworks, or technical interventions that can bring value to infertility issues phenomena. We will also explore the analogy between psychoanalytic treatment and fertility, two distinct concepts, by drawing some potential connections that can be seen as a metaphoric understanding of the therapeutic process.

Psychoanalytic understanding of psychic development

Psychoanalysis' foundations lay on Freud's discovery of the unconscious and sexuality, having the Oedipal complex and triangulation play a central role in the acceptance of the reality principle ([1875] 1975a; [1905] 1975b). Since then, there has been a shift from a model of instinctual drives to one of internal reality and objects-relations theory, and, more recently, to an intersubjectivity understanding of the treatment and to a co-construction conception of the mind. Shifting from Oedipus centrality of mental life to the emphasis given to pre-Oedipal phenomena, theorization about primitive states of mind and the importance of the mother-child relationship led to a metapsychology development with significant impacts on both practice and training. The establishment of child analysis on one hand, and setting the roots for understanding psychotic mental aspects in adults, on the other, opened the possibility to include several clinical "difficult cases", increasing both theoretical and technical basis to their analytical treatment, enabling a wider assessment of the unrepresentable in

DOI: 10.4324/9781032693446-8

ordinary people. This shaped psychoanalysis and expanded its scope of influence towards health, education, and social and cultural fields of knowledge and intervention.

One field of intervention where psychoanalysis became relevant is women's sexual health in general and fertility in particular. The wish for a child opens an original wound in the mind of each parent that will put in balance narcissistic and objectual dimensions. How does the weight of those two dimensions in this (in)fertility equation influence the path to be experienced? How does psychoanalysis apply to this specific problem?

The epistemological status in contemporary psychoanalysis establishes a casuistic order within which psychic phenomena result much more of contingency than of linear causality. We underwrite epigenetic logic, where the potentiating or inhibiting encounter between subject and object is a co-construction. Therefore, our choice is more to discuss the interconnections over infertility life stories, rather than to find an unconscious cause for them.

As a creative act, one acknowledges the presence of chaos, reparation, and reconstruction, the result of which will transform beyond expectations all parties involved. In that sense, levels of incertitude, hope and despair are brought to the stage with unpredictable outcomes. At a certain point the child, being a third, represents not only the acceptance of a stranger, but mostly the curiosity and the desire for the unknown. However, as Freud ([1919] 1975d) explained, meeting the unfamiliar always confronts us with unconscious parts of ourselves, usually related with our own *imagos* and projective identifications.

But we can also look at the psychoanalytic process according to the same premises: meeting a foreigner, crossing the borders, facing the unknown, creating new perspectives, in order to become who you really are. Therefore, how may this third party be present in psychoanalytic conceptual building? Classic drive theories relate unconscious desires and conflicts to adult sexual behavior. Object relations theory establishes how one's past experiences and attachments contribute to building identifications, fantasies, and internal object relations, which may influence the present difficulty in reproduction. Contemporary psychoanalysis, assuming a dynamic field that itself involves an analytical couple in a fertile relationship, frames the psychoanalytic process not only as a means to explore and resolve unconscious conflicts and emotional distress associated with infertility, but also as a new creative setting that combines intrapsychic with intersubjective, expanding the understanding of the emotional obstacles brought forth.

Exploring unconscious desires related to procreation, addressing the potential conflicts and repressed emotions, examining the impact of infertility on both the patient and the analyst by life storytelling recreated by the analytical couple on the setting provides unique tools that enhance the understanding and treatment of infertility towards an emotional growth experience.

Infertility experiences

What shades do infertility show in our practice? The relation between body and mind has always challenged medical practice, as well as instigated psychoanalysts to explore human development theories, in relation to which psychodynamic assessments in understanding the underlying psychosocial factors correlated seek to be found. Fertility takes a special place in this scenario and technological advances have been shaping new realities. In general, according to my clinical experience, these patients show significant signs of emotional distress, levels of frustration, anger, anxiety, depression, testifying to the implications of infertility on individuals' unfulfilled desire for parenthood. These mental processes are the angle from which the problem is about to be explored, enriched by clinical vignettes that will illustrate how this general subject may be embodied in singular life experiences and narratives and how psychoanalysis becomes the field where those dynamics are activated and transformed.

Grief and loss processes are almost automatically activated. For many, having children is a deeply rooted desire, so infertility may shatter these dreams and fantasies, leading to profound sadness, grief, and disappointment. Working through and mourning the loss of biological reproduction is immediately linked, at a mental level, with the feeling of failure specifically applied to the continuity of a personal legacy, as an unconscious defense against death anxiety, resulting in a questioning about the meaning of existence, withdrawal of libidinal investment and emotional personal crises.

For Melanie Klein (1950), every step of growth implies a mourning process (of the privileges) of the stage you left behind. Indissociable to mental primate activity, one can assume that human development's success depends on the grieving process – to be able to both lose and repair –, leading to a libidinal reinvestment in new objects and choices all throughout the life cycle. But that same ability depends, in its terms, on the quality of internal objects' representations and identifications. For Grinberg (2000), the distinction between the normal or pathological mourning process has to do with the nature of guilt involved with that particular loss: depressive guilt tends to reparation, opening the door to ambivalence; persecutory guilt compromises restoration of internal objects that become omnipresent, resisting to acknowledge separation of self-object.

Another critical psychological consequence comes from a narcissistic point of view, due to infertility's relevant impact on identity and self-esteem, self-image, and the representation of one's value. The inability to conceive or fulfill reproductive expectations may lead to experiencing feelings of inadequacy or failure. Not being able to have children might also have an impact on the way individuals perceive themselves as adult sexual beings and the intimate fulfillment of their desires, but also of their social place in a collective order. Sexual infantile fantasies and conflicts, related to love and rivalry, involved in both primary and secondary object relationship and identification process, surely play an important role in this scenario, where magical thinking, guilt, and shameful feelings, facilitated by regression, may arise and set the tone, risking to trap the individual in a traumatic situation (Alkolombre, 2008).

All these emotional reactions and clinical complaints unveil complex unconscious conflicts usually related to infantile resolutions and identifications. Freud believed that fantasies, dreams, and daydreams often reveal hidden desires and conflicts that are repressed in the unconscious mind; sexual fantasies in particular can serve as a source of psychological gratification or as a way of dealing with internal conflicts. The girl's wish for a child is originally placed at an Oedipus complex resolution, although pre-genital and anal aspects linked to primary narcissism are involved (Freud, [1917] 1975c). According to the psychosexual phallic stage, Freud argued that girls develop "penis envy", which refers to their longing for a penis due to its perception as a symbol of power and privilege. Freud proposed the concept of the "phantasy of the missing penis" which suggests that women might develop unconscious fantasies centered around compensating for their perceived lack of power or fulfilling their desires. The contribution of the classical theory's concept of penis envy to women's emotional experiences surrounding infertility interprets the inability to conceive as a metaphorical "missing phallus" relating to unconscious anxieties and desires over power, completeness, or femininity. As far as the Oedipus complex is concerned, a young girl's primary identification with her mother and, secondly, her relationship with her father, shape singular crucial dimensions to female guilt.

Moreover, fantasies around infertility might also be a way for individuals to cope with the emotions and conflicts associated with this condition. For example, women struggling with infertility might develop unconscious fantasies related to their own motherhood or the nurturing of others, which can serve as a compensatory mechanism for unfulfilled desires.

Nonetheless, Freud's work has faced significant criticism, particularly in relation to his understanding of women, and contemporaneous psychoanalysts have proposed alternative frameworks for understanding infantile sexuality and women's experiences.

Recent analysts' views helped to fill a longed-for need for both scientific and politic fairness and reliable reflection in this area, providing a distinct contribution to the psychoanalytic study of feminine psychology and sexual identity. From a comprehensive review approach on Freudian and non-Freudian views on female sexuality, several authors provided valuable understandings from a historical perspective on masculine myths about femininity and explored the origins of female narcissism. Joyce McDougall (2001), for instance, shows that female homosexuality must be integrated to achieve a harmonious feminine identity. Maria Torok (1964) gives masculinity wishes and penis envy a new role and meaning; pregnancy and uterus being seen as the equivalent of phallus symbolic representation, acknowledging in women the ability to create life with a powerful specific significance.

Cristal was a beautiful young girl when she first came to my appointment, showing signs of extreme anxiety and fear of breaking down. Soon became obvious a split in the way her mind operated, since her narrative about how she felt inside and the feedback everyone else gave her made it sound like two different people. Psychosomatic disorders, feelings of guilt and of not being enough, recurrent nightmares with explicit sexual and incestuous contents, unsuccessful love relationships, and some addictive behaviors were her frequent complaints. Despite that, she looked like a figure from a Botticelli painting, and kept talking about how wonderful her childhood had been, how admired she used to be and how lucky she had been all her life. Yet, somehow, the feeling of not deserving it all constantly remained.

In fact, right from the beginning, an unconscious fantasy less of rejection and more of not existing, nor being heard or seen, was planted in the transference-countertransference field and took shape through an enactment in which her request for consultation in my voicemail seemed to never have been noticed by me. By that I don't mean that I've forgotten it; it was more like it never had happened, since it left no trace in my memory whatsoever. As the first child, her mother, also suffering from psychosomatic diseases, had severe postpartum depression, and she described herself as a baby "permanently unsatisfied". Her aunt, but mostly her father, both played an important role. Her father, although reluctantly, took care of her, being uneasy with "feminine tasks", and being felt also as "impossible to satisfy". Curiously it took a third party (a male colleague of mine related to her) to finally bring her back to my attention and to my appointment. This enactment unveiled the nature of her drama and set the tone of how to navigate in our transference-countertransference waters.

During her first analysis, very archaic traumatic experiences became more evident, although hardly approachable. Often the session's contents were trivial, in a way that a "normality" would be a compromised solution in the sense of "this is as good as it gets". While her massive narcissistic defenses still endured, she repaired intimate relations, made important professional choices, and found meaning to her life. Having agreed on ending the process after she got married, she then said that she would most probably come back when having children would present itself as a wish. Some years later, Cristal returned, because both her aunt and father were diagnosed with cancer. She verbalized her wish of having a baby, seen as a gift to both of them. However, the idea of being infertile was present in her mind ever since she was a young girl. In fact, a period of pregnancy attempt and miscarriage occurred, that led to finding out that she was having a precocious menopause at the age of 29.

The wish for a child can be seen from different perspectives, according to some other authors. Patricia Alkolombre (2008) distinguished the "desire for a child" from the "passion for a child", highlighting in the last case strong narcissistic motivation, in a way that could be described as "a child at any cost" as in an exclusive relationship where fusional aspects of the primary idealized object seem to be at stake. Sylvie Pragier (2004) is inspired by Lacan's definition of "desire, demand or need" regarding a first diagnostic approach. The two stages in love and rivalry object choice are seen as crucial steps in a successful identification process. For both girl and boy, a complex settlement of crossed identifications takes place. First primal homosexual love towards the mother prepares a secondary unconscious identification process, which allows separation and gives access to sublimation. According to Pragier, by shifting from the mother to the father, the little girl doesn't do it because of fear of castration, as Freud's explanation goes, but because she's interested in discovering who captures mother's love and attention. Therefore, triangulation means less "with or without", than "with and without", which is a mental operation that combines love and hate through identification, providing a solution to the fear of destructiveness, rejection, and loss. Love neutralizes hate, allowing feminine and maternal to be invested all together as a result of father and mother, both narcissistic and erotic bond, which will be introjected and will play its role when the wish for a child occurs. However, in the absence of a strong enough Oedipal structure, the superego's protective role is compromised, and an ideal ego may take place, charged with demanding, and sometimes intangible, expectations and desires.

Transgenerational aspects working through projective identification transmission play their role along the way. Although reality aspects have an undoubtable effect, unconscious fantasies, within the child and both parents, keep playing an unavoidable influence. In fact, it is interesting to explore if and how new family constellations and medical assisted reproduction may preserve and transmit the core of these nuclear fantasies, and in which way do they welcome the new baby they wish for.

Fertility treatments began and the sessions were almost colonized by these persecutory fantasies focused on a body felt at war against her, as well as magical thinking used to self-punish and to confirm all her thoughts and fears.

C – I feel rotten inside; can you imagine your eggs like rotten avocados?

By doing so, on one hand apparently, she felt sadness, but, on the other, by default, she kept herself in control, not being able to access the depressive position in order to think, to mourn, to grow. In a schizoparanoid mode, she sometimes showed arrogance and contempt towards her condition and other people's empathy or tenderness. As far as transference-countertransference management is concerned, the analyst felt often trapped in an impotent, empty, unjust, and desolate environment.

C – I always said I was unable to become a mother; it's such an injustice! Screwed inheritances! Although my mom tells me: at least I made you beautiful on the outside.

A – Beautiful outside, ugly inside?

Dream: I woke up and my body had aged: I looked at myself in the mirror and I seemed to be 50-years-old and thought: I have the body of a 50-year-old woman! Life went by too fast and I didn't realize it.

At this point, a symbolic equation was the only possibility of trying to represent critical emotional experiences, resulting from unsuccessful attempts to overcome Oedipal positive identifications. To become a mother, to be like the mother/analyst, she felt cursed for feeling forced to have the same age and looks. Her wish to grow up was being punished by an internal pre-Oedipal maternal object, persecutory and retaliator, to whom she felt she had to submit.

C – My greatest disgust is not giving a nephew to my aunt; my greatest terror has always been becoming like her: bitter, alone, obese, childless; my mother gets along very well with her, but she is an unbearable person, who lives only for me and adores me and she makes a very big difference between me and my siblings which I think it's unfair; at least, at the hospital she turns life into hell to the nurses (laughs).

A – One must be entitled to hate and to protest!

Negative transference feelings were denied, but rivalry and aggressiveness towards a pre-Oedipal mother imago *grasped its way – accepted, tolerated and mitigated with compassion – in the analyst mind.*

Body and mind

One cannot approach the subject of infertility without referring to the relation between body and mind. Although we cannot establish a cause/effect on that equation, it is undeniable that emotional development has organic roots and that emotions seek bodily existence and expression. From conversive phenomena, to hypochondria, psychosomatic pathologies, or addictive behaviors, in clinical practice it is always relevant to bear in mind the moves in which unconscious conflicts express themselves through body language. Fertility and pregnancy are privileged angles to take that connection into account. Especially due to the "normality" of this life event phenomena, which puts it in a public health scale of observation and discussion.

Zygmunt Bauman (1995) notes that in societies focused on consumption the "consumer choice" is taken as an ethical value applied to any decision in life, despite all uncertainty and doubt inevitably underlying. However, if we face an universe of wide opportunities, along with the responsibility of choosing, one has to accept "the expiration date", under the risk of compromising "the embryo of the next adventure" (Bauman, 1995). Bauman sees the "logic of consumption" implicating itself in the drama of the construction of identities in the "liquid postmodernity", however, instilling in it a perennial contradiction: if, on the one hand, the perception of "being unfinished, incomplete and underutilized is a state that generates risk and anxiety", the opposite does not bring any full relief, "because it closes in advance what freedom needs to keep open" (Bauman, 1995, p. 87).

This aspect is particularly relevant if we bring into the set, on one hand, infertility issues and, one the other, medical intervention increasing the possibilities of pregnancy or parenthood. When can "primary maternal preoccupation"

(Winnicott, [1960] 1990b) arise, how may a new baby exist in this mental environment, and in which way will the mother be able to play, combining erotic and objectual bonds with her child?

In Freud's first topic ([1920] 1975e), failures at the pre-conscious function level pledged representation development. Quite often archaic traumatic experiences lead to this type of mental default. Object-relation theories, revisiting Winnicott's ideas ([1958]1990a; [1958] 1992; 1964; 1971), state that it only has psychic reality what goes through the child's experience, meaning through the process of imaginative elaboration of bodily functions. This undoubtedly finds a very clear distinction between the biological and the psychic domain. For Joyce McDougall there is a psychosomatic potential in each of us, a dimension that we keep as "exit" in the face of certain impactful affective experiences (McDougall, 2001). The body becomes a kind of stage where contemporary dramas related to identity, the meaning of life, and survival are staged; they are the "theaters of the body" (McDougall, 2000).

For Winnicott, the constitution of the third area and of the potential space (Winnicott, 1971) emerge alongside with the advent of transitional objects and the acquisition of the ability to play, presupposing a child capable of being alone. Initially in the presence of the adult and then – from the incorporation of maternal care and the constitution of the mother as a good-enough internal object – without the presence of anyone (Winnicott, 1971, pp. 31–32). Playing involves a symbolic dimension in which psychic enjoyment is greater than the physical-corporeal (p. 35). Even in the case of sexual games – in which play and sexuality come together – one could say that if the psyche does not populate the game with imaginative creations, whose enjoyment informs and sustains sexual desire, the erotic relationship will be poor and restricted. In other words, it is the ability to play that sustains sexuality, and not the other way around.

Alan Bass created the concept of "pathologies of reality" (Bass, 2000) which may also be called "normopathy". The expression refers to the subjective condition of patients who remain excessively adhered to what is shown to be real or to a specific aspect of reality. To those "concrete patients", apparently, they are quite adapted and yet, deep down, this massive adherence to a given reality represents a powerful defense against the recognition of otherness and difference. Also, we witness the disappearance of the internal world, in the sense that they function as if they do not have a psychic reality. In addition, "normopathies" illustrate one of the most common mechanisms operating on contemporary subjectivation, since over-adaptation to reality is a value in itself, promoted and incensed by medical and political narratives, with the aim of denying affections and emotions which are "not functional" to the adaptation to reality.

However, often under this "normality" a serious and potentially deadly psychic disorder is hidden: the defense against the unbearable emotions arising from a traumatic object experience forces the "normopath" to establish a radical refusal of otherness. In this way, unlike a rejection or a repression, the other becomes, for the normopath, a forever "internally lost" object. In this way, it becomes impossible to identify with the other, and all he can achieve is to measure himself with a replica of himself. The normopath is the one who experiences a constant threat to his sense of integrity and identity and the refusal of otherness is what he has left to precariously guarantee his own psychic survival. To some of these patients, one could state that aversion to the changeable character of the world is equivalent to the impossibility of playing in the Winnicottian sense (Mcdougall, 1991).

Joyce Mcdougall referred to the "anti-analysand in analysis" (Mcdougall, 1991) from clinical observations of the transferential-countertransferential dynamics of these patients that challenge the capabilities of the analyst to use it in favor of analytical work, as it is about to be presented in this work.

Cristal's aunt died before the baby was born, but the pregnancy evolved positively and a beautiful baby boy was born healthy during our summer vacations. During that time, Cristal kept sessions online and, although always planning to come and show the baby to the analyst, she never did. A very difficult period went by, both in her routines and in analysis. Taking care of him was always described as stressful, and spending time with him alone was unthinkable. Cristal was always feeling either bored, or incompetent. On one hand, Cristal was anxious for the baby to bond with her but, on the other, the fear of not being acknowledged by him as his mom, alongside with the threatening idea of being "a second choice" recurrently appeared. At the same time, the fear of not taking good care of her child was keeping her absent or distant from him, with equivalence in her avoidance coming to analysis in person, or even missing several sessions.

Up to a point Cristal confessed having been drinking and consuming drugs too much lately and being ashamed to speak about it. The analyst's intervention was based on her countertransference awareness, based on the feeling of losing place, losing sight, losing control, and having chosen to give emphasis to the helplessness within. Her not being present in sessions felt like neglect from the analyst, like if it was the analyst that wanted to keep distance from her. Cristal cried, felt very relieved and spoke about the fear of the analyst's judgment, rejection, and abandonment. For the first time in analysis, Cristal admitted how prevalent those fantasies were, but also how important the relationship with the analyst was, and gained insight on her narcissistic defenses, recovering child memories with a totally different narrative, as she had finally found and rescued the inner neglected helpless baby inside herself.

Psychoanalytic encounter as a fertility metaphor

Psychoanalysis sets a marked encounter with otherness. It takes two to create a third, but both must tolerate the unknown and overcome narcissistic obstacles. Psychoanalytic work is a chance to relive the trauma in more favorable and fertile conditions, in order to pass, through the area of experience, events that couldn't yet be reached, heard, dreamed, spoken, due to the split produced as a defense against environmental failures. Not only with the other being the patient, but mostly with those others (internal objects) within each part involved. It permanently opens a door that most likely will provide a surprise, meaning something of which there is no prior knowledge, when we least expect it, nor can it be entirely captured by the conceptual frame and yet, it challenges us beyond any expectation. Being oneself, in the presence of another, able not only to reflect, but to welcome the unknown, to resonate it within one's mind, and to be both receptive and active, to build together and help to grow something new.

Dream: I was breastfeeding, but it wasn't a baby: it was a dog or a goat: it was repulsive, but I felt obliged, because otherwise it might die. So, I thought: maybe if I step away for a while when I come back, he is already dead and there is nothing left to do…. But it wasn't like that; he was just very weak, he almost didn't move, but hopefully was still alive.

C – I saw the movie "As good as it gets". I usually don't like to watch many films, because it's hard to concentrate, but this one I liked very much. It felt nice to see how everyone struggles with their own issues but, in the end, it's the good you try to do that counts the most.

Being able to represent her terrors and bring them to the analytic setting has allowed Cristal to be able to balance fear and hope, working through and moving forward. It also brought a more alive side of her. Sessions are both more honest and pleasant and acknowledging her transferential fears of boredom, criticism, and rejection keeps us more active and fertile. Cristal's insight brought humor to the analytic relationship and, sometimes, we could laugh together. This playing ability was visible in being creative in free associations, dreams, and trivial conversations. But apparently these changes also applied to other dimensions of Cristal's life: she started to feel sick again and put on some weight … only to find out that she had gotten pregnant spontaneously.

That completely different outcome will endure, change and be changed, during the process, every single party involved. The fertility metaphor sounds entirely adequate, since receptivity to be transformed by the other in this encounter sets the requirements of a fertile ambiance where primary needs, fears, and desires arise and plant their seeds, not only to be handled and held, but primarily to be embodied, nourished, and forged into new psychic elements who will give birth to new developments of one's self. The analyst represents both a foreigner and a womb, an unsettling familiar place that invites the patient to step out of her comfort zone, to lose herself to be found, but also to find what was already potentially there. Psychoanalysis creates a third: the fertility of that unique process marks an encounter with the analyst's bisexuality and challenges both narcissistic and objectual investments to combine and to expand.

Very recently Cristal sent me, by WhatsApp, a comedian's post showing the psychoanalytic setting where the patient says: "It's still uncomfortable the idea of speaking only about me during the whole session", to which the analyst replies: "Now imagine how hard it is to only listen".

It sounded so spontaneously humble and funny, that I decided to skip neutrality and texted her back: "It's not that hard (emoji); we have endured and survived pretty well".
The following session she brought up the subject.
C – I never felt so well balanced as I feel now. I look in the mirror and although I spot the stretch marks and acne on my skin, I don't really care that much anymore, as if it makes sense, it's expected.
Her words move me and I say to her:
A – They're signs of life: you're alive Cristal! Welcome.
C – And I bring life inside of me.
Cristal thanks me while she cries.

References

Alkolombre, P. (2008). *Deseo de hijo, pásion de hijo: esterilidád y técnicas reproductivas a la luz del psicoanálisis*. Letra Viva.
Bass, A. (2000). *Difference and disavowal: The trauma of eros*. Stanford University Press.
Bauman, Z. (1995). *Modernidade e ambivalência*. Jorge Zahar.
Freud, S. ([1895] 1975a). Proyecto de psicología. In S. Freud, *Obras completas volume 1* (pp. 323–446). Amorrortu.
Freud, S. ([1905] 1975b). Tres ensayos de teoría sexual. In S. Freud, *Obras completas volume 7* (pp. 109–222). Amorrortu.
Freud, S. ([1917] 1975c). Duelo y melancolia. In S. Freud, *Obras completas volume 14* (pp. 241–255). Amorrortu.
Freud, S. ([1919] 1975d). Lo ominoso. In S. Freud, *Obras completas volume 17* (pp. 215–252). Amorrortu.
Freud, S. ([1920] 1975e). Más allá del principio de placer. In S. Freud, *Obras completas volume 18* (pp. 1–62). Amorrortu.
Grinberg, L. (2000). *Culpa e Depressão*. Climepsi Editores.
Klein, M. (1950). El duelo y su relación con los estados maníaco-depresivos. *Revista de Psicoanálisis*, 7: 415–449.
Mcdougall, J. (1991). *Em defesa de uma certa anormalidade*. Artmed. (Original work published in 1978)
Mcdougall, J. (2000). *Teatros do corpo: O psicossoma em psicanálise*. Martins Fontes. (Original work published in 1989).
Mcdougall, J. (2001). *As múltiplas faces de Eros*. Martins Fontes (Original work published in 1995).
Pragier, S. (2004). *Les bebés de l'inconscient. Le psychanalyste face aux stérilités féminines aujourd'hui*. Presses Universitaires de France.
Torok, M. (1964). La signification de l'"envie du penis" chez la femme. In J. Chasseguet-Smirgel (Ed.). *Recherches psychanalytiques nouvelles sur la sexualité féminine* (pp. 181–221). Payot.
Winnicott, D. W. (1964). *The child, the family and the outside world*. Pelican Book.
Winnicott, D. W. (1971). *Playing and reality*. Routledge.

Winnicott, D. W. ([1958] 1990a). The capacity to be alone. In *The maturational processes and the facilitating environment* (pp. 29–36). Karnac.

Winnicott, D. W. ([1960] 1990b). The theory of parent-infant relationship. In *The maturational processes and the facilitating environment* (pp. 37–55). Karnac.

Winnicott, D. W. ([1958] 1992). Primitive emotional development. In *Through pediatrics to psychoanalysis* (pp. 145–156). Karnac.

Chapter 9

The taboo of egg donation

From fairy tales to myth

Sofía Barandiaran Pérez-Yarza

The taboo of motherhood

The paper "The taboo of motherhood" (2022) is one that stems from my clinical experience with women. During my work, I have found that a common question repeats itself: why are there so many taboos surrounding motherhood? There are many subjects that people find difficult to discuss in our society in relation to conception, pregnancy and parenting, and this leads to taboos being created. These taboos, which have both a personal and a social dimension, originate from an ideal that is activated with the desire to become a mother and the frustrations that accompany such a desire. Every woman, every case of maternity or no maternity, each and every clinical case, is unique. However, it is my belief that, albeit to different degrees, they all share a common experience that is reflected in unconscious phantasies and concomitant anxieties.

I believe that thinking and speaking about these taboos may help in the elaboration process, not only in our practices but also in society, making them "less taboo" and, by so doing, alleviating the suffering. In the aforementioned paper, I analysed a number of them: the taboo of speaking about the waiting involved in order to become pregnant and the pressure that is generated internally when having to wait for a pregnancy to happen; the taboo of childbirth, associated with fear and anxiety, and the post-traumatic aftermath of that experience. Sometimes, this is reflected in clinical cases as frozen material, unspoken of and unlistened to; the taboo of miscarriage and abortion – both one's own and transgenerational – all silenced; the taboo of postnatal depression, which I consider to be underdiagnosed and insufficiently treated, as the challenges of parenthood are not sufficiently taken into account and because of the idealized portrayal of motherhood promulgating a standard of perfection; the taboo of breastfeeding, where I analysed the suffering caused by the superego imperative of breastfeeding and its vicissitudes. And the greatest taboo of them all, infertility. This chapter originates from that work and goes on to expand further the taboos surrounding assisted reproduction, and specifically egg donation.

DOI: 10.4324/9781032693446-9

I would like to summarise some of the key elements that need to be considered with regard to motherhood and the aforementioned taboos. In each woman, motherhood, as part of the feminine, is a personal and social construct derived from her internal and external experiences. The young girl, in principle, can only play with dolls; she cannot make babies. In adolescence, she will feel her body changing and her crisis regarding that great change, both physically and in terms of identity, will begin. She will be able to *make* those babies as imagined so many times. Her body will be prepared not to *play* at being mummy, but to actually *be* a mother. When she reaches adulthood, the idea of becoming a mother represents a great opportunity for the healing of narcissistic wounds, as presented by Freud in "*On narcissism: An introduction*" ([1914] 2006). The rebirth of narcissism – to love the baby as you would have wished to be loved yourself.

As the girl develops, she defers some aspects of her infantile conflict with the hope that becoming a mother will bring healing. She may say to herself: "I will not have all of my mother's love for myself. I will not have all of my father's love for myself. But I will have the most precious of all things, the baby". The phallic-Oedipal conflict, which is never completely buried, resurfaces in the woman who wishes to become a mother. Desire and, therefore, castration anxiety are activated. It may be an opportunity for narcissistic restitution, since feminine phallicism is at play (Parat, 2019). When facing motherhood, everything – the little house, the period, the womb, the ovaries, the breast – makes sense. But what drives us to seek meaning rests on a fragile narcissism, as does that of the human being, bringing us closer to what we are not. The human being finds it difficult to deal with castration – with what is lacking – and in women, if we associate castration with motherhood, if it is not "ideal, perfect, without waiting, without fears, without doubts or pain and, of course, without problems", then the idealised picture does not fit. In some cases, this may lead to much suffering, and may even call into question a woman's very existence.

In "The taboo of motherhood", I propose that a yearning for ideal fulfilment awakens in the woman who wishes to become a mother, leading us to the aforementioned taboos; those issues that women find difficult to discuss: the fears, the disappointments and the ambivalence towards the baby. Taboos are not only individual; they have a socio-cultural basis. The word "taboo" in itself expresses a conduct that is morally unacceptable in a society, group or religion. It is the prohibition of an action for an unjustified reason and based on prejudices and false beliefs. However, from a psychoanalytical perspective, we know that its justification is derived from unconscious phantasies.

Can the ideal mother be considered a religion or a belief that supports these taboos? We can observe a maternal, ancient, timeless and transgenerational ideal in, for example, the great pictorial works of Da Vinci, as discussed by Freud ([1910] 1999): *The Virgin and Child* and *The Virgin and Child with Saint Anne*. These paintings represent a Virgin mother, a mother who wants nothing more than to be a mother, the ideal mother that still resides in us all, the symbol of perfection. But she also represents a phallic mother, an almighty goddess Mut, as described by Brunswick (1940, p. 413) – "The almighty mother, capable of anything and possessor of all the attributes of pleasure".

This ideal still persists today. Contraception, career changes, the feminist struggle, the evolution of society, to mention only a few, are all factors that have contributed to women changing. They have become stronger in other facets of their lives, such as in the professional sphere. From a certain perspective, we can say that a phallic discourse has been installed – "women can be everything". This discourse may be liberating in that it allows women to be other things than just mothers. However, women may find themselves trapped in these questions – *to be or not to be, that is the question* – and the idea of the unlimited may lead to suffering.

Women, faced with the enormous challenges of today, choose to delay motherhood and disregard the passage of time, our biological finitude. They say to themselves "I, like my mother who is everything, will also be everything". From the very moment a woman decides to become a mother, the imperative of the ideal is activated – it should be now and it should be trouble-free. The difficulties a woman may encounter can be distressful and, so, the taboos emerge, such as, for example, the need to wait. It is not easy to accept that the first attempt at becoming pregnant may be unsuccessful and that it may take time. Furthermore, miscarriages, which are quite common, bring suffering. The age of maternity is a significant risk factor in miscarriages: Nybo Andersen, Wohlfahrt, Christens, Olsen & Melbye (2000) point out in their study how mothers aged 42 miscarry in more than half of their pregnancies, and women who are 45 or older have a 74.7% risk of miscarriage.

Given these problems, women can become distressed and often experience high levels of anxiety when they begin fertility treatments. Current guidelines for treatments in the Spanish national health service (BOE n° 269)[1] recommend trying naturally for one year after the age of 30 and, if unsuccessful, to then commence treatment.

Treatment will usually start with insemination and, if that does not go well, it will continue with *in vitro* procedures. Assisted reproduction is, undeniably, an important step forward. But it may also bring with it great suffering. Women endure profound anxiety during the procedures, which are neither easy nor painless. They submit their bodies to hormones, surgery, anaesthetics, but that is not all: they also experience illusion and disillusionment. A great many women suffer the unspeakable after a succession of *in vitro* cycles. Nobody helps them to stop or take a break because the possibility of failure has been relegated. I believe there are many factors at play here; one that may be considered is the impossibility of dealing with failure, seemingly so painful that the woman would rather suffer the other physical and emotional pains, dreadful as they are, but apparently more bearable. Each unsuccessful attempt brings with it considerable grief. However, there can be no time to complain or mourn: the urge will push them onwards towards trying again. But from what are they fleeing? From the great taboo – infertility: not to be a mother may imply not to be a woman, and this is precisely the greatest fear – to be nothing.

Another key point to consider in order to understand the challenges of motherhood, both with regard to assisted and unassisted reproduction, is the relationship between the woman and her own mother: the so-desired mythical reunion with her, and the hostility and guilt felt for failing to be like her; in ART this may be reflected in her difficulty to become a mother.

For a better understanding of this relationship with the mother, let us examine its source – the girl inside the woman. In her theory, Klein ([1932] 1997) proposes the idea of the primitive maternal imago of the nourishing breast, the father's penis, the children and the power to satisfy all needs. This all-powerful figure generates frustration in the child and may give rise to envy, anger and attacks towards the breast and the mother's internal body in her phantasy. When that is the case, retaliation will return in the same way. Castration anxieties[2] in women may lead to phantasies of damage to the internal body, to her reproductive function and, also, to her potential babies. Having a child subdues these anxieties, lending hope to the possibility of having good internal objects, whilst the adversities reactivate the anxiety of having destroyed them.

The obstacles that must be overcome during the process of trying to become a mother call into question the entire essence of the female being. The most primitive phantasy once again comes into play. The all-powerful imago seems to be reactivated and, with it, the frustration of not fulfilling it. The illusion of the fairy tale (being a perfect mother) becomes disillusionment and may transform into the tragedy that we find in myths.

The taboo of egg donation

Having introduced the issues at stake when a woman wishes to become a mother and the taboos, phantasies and emotions involved when faced with difficulties, I would now like to focus on the taboos in assisted reproduction, especially with regard to egg donation. A woman must renounce the possibility of becoming a mother using her own eggs and must embrace the idea of having eggs donated. I say "embrace" because if one cannot embrace, contain and elaborate the psychological work required, the myth might tragically unfold.

In general, when a woman or a couple reach the egg donation stage, they have already been riding the roller coaster of illusion-disillusionment for quite some time. Each attempt brings with it illusion and each failure brings disillusionment. The erotic portrayal has long disappeared, cooled down, become lost in the medical examinations, the ultrasounds, the hormones, the inseminations, the punctures, the beta-waits and the grief. The narcissistic questioning at this point is often devastating. A woman might wonder: What is wrong with me? What don't I have? What's at fault? What am I lacking? What haven't I been given to be a woman, to be a mother? Am I not woman enough? – this is a tale of guilt – Have I killed it? – after a negative result following treatment – Perhaps I don't want it? What am I doing wrong? Who has the defect, me or my partner?[3]

In the consulting room, we often find that frustrated desire can transform into anger and guilt, and unconscious phantasies are put into motion. Repression is no longer functioning efficiently and the ego finds itself overwhelmed with primitive and, sometimes, fierce anxieties. The woman may become de-identified, weak, lonely, angry, destructive and, at the same time, destroyed.

The identifying fabric that supports her ego can become loose. She may feel de-identified from her own emotions and their intensity. It is not uncommon to witness a woman weep bitterly as a reaction to the news of a friend's pregnancy and to feel as if she were the worst person in the world for her reaction. There may be feelings of hatred towards the internal parental couple, projected on the pregnant women she sees in the streets, the number of which seem to have suddenly multiplied! She may feel miserable and guilty, and disillusionment reigns. At times, her anger may allow her to become detached – a defence mechanism against depression. What I call the "karmic blame game" intensifies, as she searches for an explanation for what is happening to her. Her experiences and the decisions she may have taken in the past return with a burden of guilt; her abortion during adolescence; not having tried to conceive earlier – all are possible hypotheses for the difficulties she encounters. The burden causes stress as she faces a great fear. In the words of Klein ([1932] 1997) the "girl's deepest fear – namely that the inside of her body has been injured or destroyed and that she has no children or only damaged ones" (p. 210).

Every decision in assisted reproduction comes with a series of concomitant phantasies and, therefore, every step taken by a couple in assisted reproduction should allow sufficient time for elaboration. These couples need to deal with grief, but this becomes difficult when they are oppressed by time. Sometimes, the distress is so overwhelming that steps are taken without enough thought and depressive feeling brings on fear. Thus, one rushes forward. The analyst may find it hard to set up the conditions for a psychotherapeutic process and, in this respect, assisted reproduction clinics are, at times, unhelpful by exerting pressure. However, the possibilities of representation and elaboration of every step in the process and its vicissitudes will be crucial, as we will see in the clinical vignettes.

It is in this context that the donation of gametes comes into the picture. Questions arise: Is this ethical? Why would a woman do this, donate her precious eggs? Out of altruism? And what if she is impulsive and in the future she can't have babies and she regrets what she has done? And what if the child searches for her? Is this legal? Egg donation gives rise to phantasies such as the stealing of eggs from another woman; the taking away of children from another. We can approach an understanding of the density of the conflict through McDougall (1999), who speaks about "the phantasised stealing from the mother of the essence of her femininity" (p. 285). But, we can also deepen our understanding through the myths of witches and fairies, such as the *lamiak* in the Basque Country, who would take children from their homes, as we will see later.

Who is the mother? The difficulties of disclosure

With respect to the legal regulations that control egg donation, there are differences between countries. In Spain, egg donation is confidential and only legal if made altruistically, with financial compensation given only for the trouble taken regarding the process. In the USA, there is a supply of donors, where one may choose from catalogues showing success records and prices. Each option unleashes different phantasies. In Spain, donations are anonymous and in France they are not, but, interestingly, practices in Spain are full of French women. We have to consider the questions that may be at play: rivalry with the donor; wishing and not wishing to know the identity of the donor; the possibility, or impossibility, of accepting something so vital from another woman.

One might also consider unresolved genetic grief. When a woman is to have a baby conceived through egg donation, there is a grieving process as she will not be able to share her genes with the embryo and, as a consequence, concerns arise. What if it doesn't look like me? What if the child is too unfamiliar, too dissimilar? When one is unable to elaborate this grief, a solution may be found in the form of denial. In Spain, patients are sometimes medically advised *not* to disclose, neither to the child nor to the relatives, that the child does not originate from the patient's gametes. This may result in internal denial and hinder the elaborative work required.

However, in my clinical experience, although it cannot be generalised, it is not uncommon to find that patients choose not to follow this medical advice. In other words, they decide to disclose. Indeed, there are parents who attend our practices in order to seek guidance on how to disclose such information to their children. Freeman-Carroll (2016), in her article on this subject, highlighted the difficulties of parental disclosure to offspring conceived through oocyte donation: the intention to do so *versus* reality. Many families unwittingly do not follow through with their original plans to disclose. In my opinion, and based on my clinical experience, disclosure, from a psychoanalytic perspective, makes sense, since the secrecies of filiation tend to be pathogenic secrecies.

Disclosure brings with it further questions for the parents. In the following vignette, we can see what may be at play. In a recent interview, a single mother revealed her concerns to me. Her son, who was four-years-old, would ask her all types of questions in relation to the pregnancy. He would ask her how long he had been in her tummy, when he would breastfeed. The mother was unsure of how to approach this questioning. He had been born through surrogacy and using the egg from another woman. She had always wished to tell her son the truth, but she had become paralysed with the idea that this would destroy him. This led me to ask myself who would be destroyed: the son or the mother herself, on revealing the truth, on showing him her non-mother side, on revealing her injury? She came to me for help with disclosure. How could she tell her son that there existed another mummy? Was she herself a mummy? She was faced with difficult concerns and was troubled by her anxieties. Despite these concerns, she did not wish to commence psychotherapy for herself but she *did* request professional advice from an analyst on how to tell her son. By doing so, she was able to share her fears and understood that her own elaboration of the process was perhaps intervening when she considered the information to be destructive for her son. This calmed her and helped her to continue with her wish to share her story with her son and, thus, not create a taboo.

Martha and the *Lamiak* – between the destructive mother and Mother Earth

In order to approach an understanding of the anxiety suffered by the woman in the previous vignette, let us consider what unconscious phantasies we may be dealing with. I would like to introduce Martha. She has helped me to address two issues that I have observed in other patients; the way in which the ideal with respect to motherhood has the capacity to oppress, and the impact of the "competition-related vertigo", stimulated by the Oedipus conflict and its aspect of rivalry with the mother, as described by Quinodoz (2003, p. 1).

During Martha's analysis, we began to understand an ambivalent relationship with an idealised and disappointing mother. Years before beginning analysis, she had already decided to become a mother. For her, becoming a mother would bring her closer to the ideal that "to be a mother would be to know everything", an idealisation on which we worked. We could also see how the phantasy of being a mother herself evoked taking the place of her own mother and taking her mother's babies. This unsettled her.

When she made the decision to become a mother, she had to endure successive difficulties that connected her to the frustrations of motherhood – frustrations she now embodied. She suffered a miscarriage, which caused her great distress, given that she had not expected so many things to go wrong. She felt her inner self was dead with nothing more to offer; something lifeless, destroyed. This reminded me of Quinodoz (2003) and her work on how the female body can be represented and, specifically, how the female genitals may be seen as a "lifeless thing-like container" (p. 8). Martha felt her entire being was in question. It became apparent that the guilt felt for her desires was related to the "amputation anxiety" (p. 11) of her female organs and her childbearing capacity; she felt that her ability to "contain" was damaged.

Martha became pregnant again and started to feel a disturbing aggressiveness towards her mother. She felt misunderstood; she thought that her mother was stealing her limelight, and that she would eventually steal her baby. Her mother was excited, perhaps one could say even manically so, at the thought of having a grandchild. But she did not identify with her daughter's distress. For Martha, it was as if her mother wanted the child for herself and she feared that she would become a bad and incapable mother and, so, the grandmother would entice the baby; steal the baby. There were other women in her life that triggered similar phantasies. She felt that they had the capacity to "take away her child" because the child would not love her and because she would be unable to handle and contain the child. During analysis, we were able to see that her desire to be a mother was punished in her phantasy with the incapacity to *become* a mother; she felt that miscarriage was her punishment.

Then, something happened. It was Saint John's Eve, an important day in the Basque Country, a magical night. On this night, bonfires are lit, reminiscent of times when witches were burnt. In Basque folklore there is a plethora of witch tales, magical and powerful women, such as the goddess Mari, symbolic of a matriarchal system. It was on this night that her mother gave her an *eguskilore*.

The *eguskilore* – which can be translated as flower of the sun – is a rare, large flower which grows high up in the mountains and is hung on the entrance doors of *caseríos* (typical Basque farmhouses) for protection. I was unaware of the legend about which she spoke. The *eguskilore* were presented as gifts by *Amalur* (which means Mother Earth) as protection during the dangerous nights when the *lamiak* (evil spirits) would walk from house to house searching for babies to steal. If there was an *eguskilore* hanging on the door, the *lamiak* would have to stop to count the enormous number of petals on the flower and dawn would come well before the spirit had completed the count. It was very symbolic and reassuring for Martha to think that her mother was giving her protection, and this brought her closer to *Amalur* – Mother Earth – to the good mother and to the sensation of retrieving her good internal objects. This helped her to repair the image she had of her mother and, thus, that of herself as a mother. In our sessions, she considered the receiving of the *eguskilore* as the granting of permission. Being able to elaborate these phantasies of competition and of stealing helped her to process her fears and to internally connect with her potential to be a good mother.

Martha's case helped me to identify these phantasies in other cases and relate them to cases on which I was working with respect to women who were having difficulties conceiving. I became interested in the malicious facet of the *lamiak*. I had previously considered them to be exquisite creatures living close to the rivers, breathtakingly beautiful. I imagined them as the fairies from tales of old, but I began to research their dark side; a seductive-murderous side with men and robbers of children in order to devour them. The fairy becomes a witch. How did this monstrosity come to be? During the course of my research, I encountered the myth of Lamia (interestingly, similar in name).

Lamia was the daughter of King Belus of Egypt and Lybie. She was a princess of great beauty and loved by the God of Gods, Zeus. However, a terrible tragedy would occur. Hera, the wife of Zeus, reacted with rage upon learning of the romance between her husband and Lamia. In revenge, Hera harmed the children of Lamia. According to some versions, she took them and killed them. In others, she forced Lamia to kill them herself. This drove her insane and she began to snatch babies from mothers who were more fortunate than her, in order to devour them. Her terrifying acts transformed the once beautiful princess into a monster.[4]

The myth of the beautiful princess converted into a child-devouring monster elicits thought-provoking questions. If we analyse this, in the myth there is a daughter, a princess chosen by Zeus (father), fulfilling her Oedipal desire, one might think. This leads to the appearance of the enraged woman-wife of Zeus, Hera, who punishes her by taking away her children. Lamia had stripped her of her place and would receive punishment for this act. In psychoanalysis we see that this punishment is for the fulfilment of desire. "Your children will die, you will become insane" – perhaps two of the greatest fears for a woman going through assisted reproduction procedures, the inability to have children and the fear of becoming insane.

Let us return to our fairy tale, to the princess, to her illusions; a woman longing for children who, at the time, was trying to fulfil her childhood desire of being like her mummy, of having babies like her. What is the fairy tale? In the psychosexual development of girls, that which is latent – because the Oedipus complex is not entirely buried – is the double primo Oedipal desire: to be everything *for* the mother and to be everything *with* the mother, or, if not, to be like the mother and conquer a different object – the father – who will give her that even more precious object, the baby. The moment arrives: she is on the starting line – like Cinderella, accompanied by her fairy godmother and heading towards her Prince Charming – to fulfil her transformed desire, to live her own tale. The accompaniment of the fairy godmother could depict what is lovingly given by the mother: her permission to be a woman, to grow up.

But, in tales, we also find the wicked – the step-mothers, the step-sisters – representing envy, attack, rivalry, fratricide. The most primitive phantasy is at play. To exceed the mother and take her place as a "mother" is an aspect of growing up. It is something to elaborate at an unconscious level and generates conflict. Electra[5] appears and, with her, the phantasies: committing matricide, being the one that seduces the father, the one that has the child, being the mother, being more than the mother, potentially evoking a destructive aspect of rivalry with the mother. To occupy that desired place is conflictive because it may equate with killing the mother in the phantasy; hurting her, or taking her place.

If we turn back to the subject of ART, when there is no pregnancy, as indicated earlier, the woman questions herself at the deepest level. In some cases, it may seem that there is no opportunity for sublimation and the Lamia fairy is at risk of feeling she is becoming the Lamia monster and may even incarnate her. The connection with the destructive and aggressive aspect of rivalry is crude as it connects with unconscious phantasies.

The tragic side: The myth

To provide an insight into the darkness of the myth, I would like to present a brief clinical vignette. Some years ago, I received in my practice a six-year-old boy, conceived through egg donation. The sperm was from the father. They were an older couple and had come because of the boy's bad behaviour at home. I emphasise *at home* because it was *there* that they were all infuriated and the parents were unable to impose limits.

I began to evaluate the boy and to work with him. In the absence of his mother's gaze, he was different. On working with the parents, I was able to make sense of what was contained in that look. In the boy, the mother saw the donor who, in her imagination, was a psychopath and mentally ill. The gaze was quasi-delusional and could not be amended. This made me wonder: who was the Lamia? The donor, as projected by the recipient? Or the recipient, a woman who was unable to process a part of her castration, the impossibility of having children and who, in her phantasy, felt she had resorted to stealing something from another woman? This consideration was so unsettling that, in the absence of the possibility of elaborating, it remained trapped, frozen in her gaze.

My work with the boy proceeded well. A key aspect was the work on his identity as a good son or bad son. For the parents, to see the bad son as the son of the donor split away from the good son, so desired by them, was also fruitful. The parents were able to understand the dynamics at play and position themselves differently. They became lovingly closer and the son responded. The mother refused treatment but *did* understand, to a certain degree, how her gaze was influencing her son. From her maternal side within, she became more relaxed, helping her to grow closer to her son. However, the mother's gaze never profoundly changed. Something was trapped in that look. She could still observe a psychopathic potential in him and the risk of becoming mentally ill. As an afterthought, I pondered the unthinkable regarding this case, giving me cause to question the difficulty in elaborating the origin of her son.

Lamia – bogey-woman versus Lamia – Mother Earth

The idea of the Lamias, the bogey-women, seems to be universal and may be a phantasy to elaborate within each woman during the egg donation process. But, also, every woman must elaborate the destructive side of the feminine identity – a wicked witch, a thief, like the one in the story of Hansel and Gretel; the witch that kidnaps children and prods them with her stick to see if they are ready enough to be devoured. In different cultures we see how myths and customs that reflect these phantasies are repeated. On discussing this work, a Turkish colleague, Melis Tanik Sivri (personal communication), introduced me to a custom in her country where women are not permitted to be alone for a period of time after giving birth, as if there was a fear that someone might come to take away the baby. In Mexico, women tie a red string bracelet to their babies to ward off negative vibes and misfortune brought about by the evil eye. In Greece, the country where the Lamia myth originates, the figure of the bogey-woman that takes away children (as opposed to the bogey-man in other cultures) is used to frighten children. Most likely, if we take the time to investigate ancient beliefs in each country, we might discover similar references in relation to the fear of a woman who becomes insane and hurts and robs the children of others.

Recently, in my hometown, a newborn baby was kidnapped from a hospital. This was talked about in the news and in social circles for weeks. Some talked about the terrible witch that should be imprisoned. For others, she was a poor, sick woman who was unable to realise her project and had had to fake her pregnancy and then enter a hospital to steal a baby. This led me to consider what it is that creates the notion of a woman who kidnaps children and I asked myself: how does a woman who must turn to egg donation in order to become a mother elaborate the phantasy of being a bogey-woman?

In a short story that I have used as material in egg donation cases, *"Un Regalo de Vida Chiquitito"* by Martinez (2011, *A Tiny Itsy Bitsy Gift of Life*), the portrayal of the donor seemed interesting. An older female rabbit, surrounded by little rabbits, comes to give a small seed to a young female rabbit who cannot be a mother. This made me reflect on the possibility of seeing the donor as a mother figure; a donor of attributes.

Indeed, it is my belief that egg donation can only be accepted if regarded as protection by *Amalur* (Mother Earth). When a woman is faced with egg donation, after asking herself many questions and trying to elaborate them, a good female figure must reappear in her mind: a woman who donates her products because she is able to share, because she is gifted and *wants* to give.

Another one of my patients had tried various, unsuccessful, ART cycles when she began psychotherapy. She was doubtful as to whether to try again, but decided to do so, and failed. Then, the idea of egg donation occurred. This idea had, for some time, worried and depressed her. What particularly unsettled her was the idea of the donor regretting her decision, or that the child would search for her. She was haunted by questions such as whether she would be capable of making the child "her own". She feared that the child would not look like her and questioned the ethics of the procedure. After much reflection on the subject of egg donation and working through her unconscious phantasies, she told me: "I was visited by my niece, who is studying medicine, and she thought it was beautiful that there existed donors and added that she would like to become one. I thought about this, and I now believe that if I had known about this possibility while at university, I would have donated". With this reassuring notion in mind, together with all the previous elaborative work we had undertaken, she decided to commence the egg donation process.

This good mother-daughter dyad incarnated into the niece who can offer her phallic gifts, because there is love to give, filled her with hope and she began to see egg donation in a different light. I believe that, within her, being able to connect to that which is donated by parents who are sufficiently complete, from a narcissistic perspective, capable of letting the child go – as described by Bergeret (1975) – allowed her to connect with the woman-mother who was able to donate her eggs. This permitted her to use those gifts and helped her in her decision to walk the path – a fairy godmother, an internal mother, representing the woman who lets the child go, with a triangular function in her mind; a woman for whom her children are independent beings and not a narcissistic prolongation. She represents a benevolent figure that one may identify with and that must exist internally, otherwise she will find it difficult to connect.

But why is it so important to have and to reunite with the good internal objects, with the fairy godmother? It is important in order to be able to cope with the ominousness of the experience. Pregnancy must be embraced both physically and mentally. One must embrace this little alien, which is the "I" but also the "Not-I", growing inside. For a woman, when everything has taken place internally, inside her body, it will, generally, be easier for her to tolerate what is external to her. But a woman who has received the donation of eggs may find the elaboration of her phantasies a difficult challenge. This is crucial in order for her to accept the embryo and, in turn, the child.

It is not uncommon to find women who, without having elaborated the different stages, become pregnant and feel rejection. We must, therefore, consider that risk.[6] When this is the case, guilt returns and the internal baby-object might turn into a bad, invasive parasitic object, which may be felt as damaging, or damaged, as reflected in the phantasies described. There is anxiety that it will come out "bad", as we have seen in the clinical case of the six-year-old boy discussed earlier; like a "poisonous excrement" as described by Klein ([1932] 1997). Or that the child will not do well in life and so the ideal will not be fulfilled. This can happen in the case of any child, regardless of their origin. The infantile phantasy of harming the mother's body may have been reactivated and, in revenge, "their mother will attack and despoil it (her body) and will put 'bad' things inside it in exchange for the 'good' ones" (p. 209). In any woman, motherhood has the potential for disordering as well as ordering. What was constructed is at risk of becoming de-constructed. The most primitive phantasy may invade the woman's mind and the child may suffer a distressing overload. Let us not forget what Klein proposes: for a woman, her child becomes "the embodiment of her own ideals which she has not been able to attain and, through her child, she will replicate both her good and her bad experiences with her objects" (p. 228). Without doubt, a considerable amount of psychological work is required.

The mother receiving an egg must be able to feel a part of *herself* in the baby. Recent research (Xavier, Roman, Aitken & Nixon, 2019) shows how the mother can influence embryonic gene expression causing epigenetic change. The mother may perceive this idea as a way of influencing the baby and, thus, passing on a part of herself. It is something that may provide her with reassurance. This might allow her to bond with the other being; a bonding with that which has been provided by the couple or by the male or female donor. The mother must be able to internally reproduce a triangular scene where she is the daughter of parents who love each other and, in turn, this will give rise in her to a child who can be loved. It must be a mix in which her ego is not suffocated, where incestuous wishes do not annul her ego; an epigenetic mix that transmits genetic information and phantasies between the donor, the pregnant mother and the baby. One must be able to tolerate and bear this, whilst finding the beauty in creation and in sublimation.

Conclusions

Motherhood calls into question the female being as a whole and it is for this reason that so many taboos exist surrounding this subject. Each and every woman, in a unique way, must deal with the immense amount of elaboration required for the choices she makes in life: maternity, no maternity, ART, surrogacy, adoption.... Clinical work enables us to focus on certain forms of elaboration and allows us to analyse the unconscious phantasies that may be at play. Assisted reproduction is a relatively new element that will awaken unconscious phantasies already considered in psychoanalytic theory. However, it is my belief that it is now the task of psychoanalysts to take another look in order to gain a deeper understanding.

My clinical work has enabled me to observe how egg donation gives rise to phantasies such as the stealing of eggs from another woman; the taking away of children from another. Interestingly, by looking at myths and folklore, we can find material to help us understand the unconscious phantasies with which we are dealing. Myths and stories of witches, such as the *Lamiak* in the Basque Country, help us to connect with the destructive and aggressive feelings of rivalry, reactivated by frustration and grief. Working through these phantasies, we have seen how fairy tales and fairy godmothers are needed in order to placate those feelings of rivalry. The fairy godmother, Mother Earth, all of these are good internal objects with which the patient must connect in order to embrace, contain and elaborate the psychological work required and bond with the child.

In this chapter, I have introduced the reader to a number of women and their stories, all of them trying to take control of their frustration depending on their elaborative capacity; beautiful lamias that sense that, in their madness, they are becoming bogey-women; robbers of babies.

I have presented the taboo of egg donation and related it to other taboos regarding motherhood in order to reflect on the phantasies that might awaken, so we are able to accompany these women and, whenever possible, elaborate that bond of filiation and, thus, not encounter tragedies.

Notes

1 BOE Boletín Oficial del Estado. Official State Gazette (Spain).
2 I use the term "castration anxiety" as defined by Klein: "The girl's very intense anxiety about her womanhood can be shown to be analogous to the boy's dread of castration, for it certainly contributes to the checking of her Oedipus impulses" (Klein, [1928] 1992, p. 195).

3 I will not be focussing here on the crisis in the couple nor on the man's suffering. However, it is important to note that the man's suffering and his exclusion are also important issues.

4 https://es.wikipedia.org/w/index.php?title=Lamia&oldid=149801434.

5 Electra, daughter of King Agamemnon, murders her mother in order to avenge the death of her father. Jung ([1912] 2000) describes the Electra complex as the love of a daughter towards her father leading to competition with her mother, considering her a rival. The girl fears losing her mother's love, which helps her to identify herself with her own mother.

6 Likewise, it should be noted that such a feeling of rejection may also occur with women who become pregnant "naturally".

References

Barandiaran, S. (2022). El tabú de la maternidad. *Revista de psicoanálisis de la Asociación Psicoanalítica de Madrid*, 95: 423–445.

Bergeret, J. (1975). *Manual de psicología patológica*. Editorial Ilustrada.

Brunswick, R. (1940). La fase preedípica del desarrollo de la libido. *Revista de psicoanálisis argentina*, 1 (3): 403–426.

Freeman-Carroll, N. (2016). The possibilities and pitfalls of talking about conception with donor egg: Why parents struggle and how clinicians can help. *Journal of Infant, Child and Adolescent Psychotherapy*, 15 (1): 40–50.

Freud, S. ([1910] 1999). Un recuerdo de Leonardo da Vinci. In *Obras completas volume 11* (pp. 53–129). Amorrortu.

Freud, S. ([1914] 2006). Introducción al narcisismo. In *Obras completas volume 14* (pp. 65–98). Amorrortu.

Jung, C. ([1912] 2000). Ensayo de exposición de la teoría psicoanalítica. Sobre psicoanálisis. In *Obra completa volume 4* (pp. 150–151) Trotta.

Klein, M. ([1928] 1992). Early stages of the Oedipus conflict. In *Love, guilt and reparation and other works* (pp. 186–198). Karnac.

Klein, M. ([1932] 1997). *The psycho-analysis of children*. Vintage.

Martinez, C. (2011). *Un regalo de vida chiquitito (A tiny itsy bitsy gift of life)*. Jover.

McDougall, J. (1999). Sobre la homosexualidad femenina. In J. Chasseguet-Smirgel (Ed.), *La sexualidad femenina* (pp. 243–299). Biblioteca Nueva.

Nybo Andersen, A., Wohlfahrt, J., Christens, P., Olsen, J. & Melbye, M. (2000). Maternal age and foetal loss: population based register linkage study. *BMJ*, 320 (7251): 1708–1712. DOI: 10.1136/bmj.320.7251.1708

Parat, C. (2019). Lo fálico femenino. *Revista de psicoanálisis*, 87: 717 – 738.

Quinodoz, D. (2003). A particular kind of anxiety in women. In M. Alizade (Ed.), *Studies on femininity* (pp. 1–14). Karnac.

Xavier, M., Roman, S., Aitken, R. & Nixon, B. (2019). Transgenerational inheritance: how impacts to the epigenetic and genetic information of parents affect offspring health. *Human Reproduction Update*, 25(5): 518–540. DOI: 10.1093/humupd/dmz017

Chapter 10

Symbolic affiliation in a case of egg donation

Renata Viola Vives

"He is not my son" – On an egg donation case

This chapter deals with a clinical case of a nine-year-old boy, the result of an egg donation, whose school difficulties led his mother to seek analysis. During Gabriel's story, a narrative emerges in which the mother did not recognize him as a son, as he was the result of a donated egg. From this narrative and fragments of the boy's analytic sessions, it is possible to reflect on how assisted reproduction technologies create new questions about the concept of motherhood, for example, as Fiorini (2001) tells us, and can also lead to scarce possibilities of psychic inscription. In the clinical case, the non-recognition of Gabriel's symbolic affiliation or symbolic non-adoption seems to have interfered with his psychic constitution, creating great obstacles to his development, aspects that were allied to the secrecy regarding the origin (egg donation). All these aspects may have led to the creation of representational failures and inhibition for learning, characteristics that Gabriel presented.

As Fiorini (2001) points out, since the origins of culture there has never been any doubt about what it is to be a mother, where certainties about motherhood have always been opposed to doubts about fatherhood. Currently, however, assisted reproduction technologies have begun to challenge these certainties, causing psychoanalysts to ask several questions concerning motherhood, fatherhood, and filiation. The concepts of motherhood and fatherhood are combined with the possibility of postponing motherhood and even the decision not to be a mother, in some women.

In this context, Fiorini (2001) tells us about the need to differentiate reproduction and motherhood, considering that the former is of the "natural" order, while the latter implies a human experience, where love, desire, creativity, the body, and its representation are intertwined.

These ideas are supported by the contributions of Badinter (1980) when she states that maternal love does not correspond to an innate feminine tendency, but that it depends to a large extent on a variable behavior according to the culture and customs of the time, stating that there is a variability of maternal feeling, according to the ambitions or frustrations of the mother in each culture.

DOI: 10.4324/9781032693446-10

However, throughout their lives, many women, when they wish to have children, will face the momentary or definitive impossibility of fulfilling this desire, facing infertility. Infertility, in culture, is compared to disability, to a dry woman or even to "not being a woman", and in men it is synonymous with impotence, with little virility. For these situations, but not only for them, reproductive technologies will emerge, that is, the medical-technological intervention will present itself to carry out pregnancies that would not happen spontaneously.

For some of these cases of infertility, the indication will end up being the reception of gametes, such as eggs. When the treatment refers to eggs received, sometimes we see a difficulty of the mother in connecting with the child.

In any case, all these technological advances raise ethical, legal, and psychological questions. Assisted fertilization with one's own gametes, the freezing of eggs or embryos, gestation by surrogacy, semen banks, embryo donation, egg donation, twin pregnancies, pregnancy losses, and prematurity are all solutions or consequences of medicine, but they are not always psychically inscribed experiences, sometimes with few possibilities for processing and subjectivizing inscriptions.

Would the very question of infertility be one of the experiences that might not be psychically inscribed to the point where we can ask ourselves which infertility we are talking about, infertility of the body or psychic infertility? Here we are thinking of psychic infertility as the impossibility of psychically sheltering a baby, the impossibility of assuming another place in the generational chain, as well as the impossibility of symbolically adopting a child.

Next, we will present the clinical case of Gabriel, who came in for analysis due to several symptoms related to school issues. At the very beginning of his treatment, in the interviews with the mother, she reveals that she does not recognize him as a son, because he was the product of an egg donation.

Gabriel is nine years old and has been referred for a psychodiagnostic evaluation: he presents depressive traits, psychomotor difficulties, and self-esteem issues, with an IQ above average. He presents school difficulties, has difficulty concentrating, and has difficulties in the area of languages, as he cannot "write stories". His texts have no punctuation, paragraph, beginning, middle, or end.

In the first interview, the mother, Paula, comes alone. She says she is separating from Paulo, Gabriel's father, because he is "not morally reliable", and the couple also has financial problems. They had been separated for about a month, but they stayed in the house and soon reconciled. When the analyst asked what her husband's issues were, she was a little evasive, saying that he did not follow rules, doing what suited him and that worried her a lot. She said that she had told her husband that she was coming and asked him to come to the session, but Paulo didn't show up. Paula told little about the family history, dwelling more on Gabriel's symptoms.

When Paula arrived at the second interview, she immediately said:

P: I have to tell you something: He's not my son.

Paula's speech ended up causing great surprise to the analyst, who did not understand what the boy's mother was talking about. When encouraged to speak, she reaffirmed: "He is not my son, because he comes from a donated egg".

Paula then reported that she separated from her first husband at the age of 32, when she became a director of a large company and had to move to another city; she was on her own taking care of the couple's son, João. She met Paulo soon after the divorce and they began a relationship. He had no children and, according to her, Paulo really wanted to be a father. They tried the natural method and were unsuccessful; they went for *in vitro* fertilization and were unsuccessful; she had an early menopause, when she discovered that her eggs were not viable, and was recommended fertilization with egg donation.

Paula seemed indifferent in her speech, not expressing any emotion. At the same time, she seemed like a very "dedicated" mother, extremely worried about Gabriel. She took care of her son's school tasks and sought his good school performance, which seemed to be her biggest concern. She said that Gabriel did not know about the egg donation and this should remain "secret". She had actually gotten out of control with Paulo when he had told Gabriel.

P: He could never have told. What's going to change? I didn't authorize him to tell. If he had a serious illness he needed to know about, that's fine. But he has the same blood type as us, so he wouldn't be suspicious. Paulo could not have told.

Paulo and Gabriel were watching TV when a program about assisted reproduction came on. Paulo looked at Gabriel and said that he had been born this way, from *in vitro* fertilization, that there were three babies, and that Gabriel was the only one left. Gabriel asked him if he had killed his brothers. Paulo said no more.

For Tubert (1996), the couple will configure their desire to have a child from the fall of their narcissistic omnipotence and the acceptance of castration. A man and a woman's desire for a child arises when both recognize that they need each other, not to achieve wholeness, but as partners in precariousness, in flaw. In this way, the couple manages to invest a necessary space to receive the baby, giving him a symbolic place and including him in a generational chain. Every child needs to be adopted symbolically.

Mann (2018) states that unconscious fantasies play an important role before conception, during pregnancy, and postpartum and affect feelings towards the child. Many questions arise, especially about the psychic consequences on individuals and the result of these technologies, that is, the child to come, especially in cases of egg donation. So, what fantasies would have dominated Paula, from the moment she discovered herself infertile until the indication of egg donation? And how would she have experienced the pregnancy?

Faria (2005) states that the woman who receives donated eggs may present anxiety that when the child is born, he will physically resemble another woman.

This other woman could be considered a rival and, in this sense, "more of a woman", more fertile, because she would be able to give life. The recipient might be distressed at the thought, "What will it be like when they ask me who the baby looks like?"

Another unbearable fantasy for the woman who receives donated eggs, according to Faria (2005), is that the child will feel more like the son of the genitor/father than of herself, feeding a doubt: "Will he like his father more than me?"

Paula had stated in the interviews:

P: Sometimes I wonder if this can be a problem, him not having my genetics. I don't think so, because João is physically similar to me and Gabriel is with his father, because he is very similar to his father, so it's okay, everything is sorted out.

Was the issue of genetics so well resolved for this woman, if at the same time, she affirmed that Gabriel was not her son, despite having gestated and cared for him for nine years? Or did the affirmation of the resemblance between father and son express her anguish at thinking Gabriel was more connected to his father than to herself? Could it have been these fantasies that would have led to the couple's separation? To divorce?

The egg, then the embryo, needs to gain body in the phantasmatic tissue of the mother so that she can adopt it symbolically. When the baby is born, however, he may still be felt as a stranger.

The birth of a baby can also mean a place of lesser value for the woman and can reinforce the couple's estrangement, as well as intensify severe paranoid fantasies and situations of rejection of the child. Faria (2005) highlights some aspects of each trimester during pregnancy in women who received donated eggs, especially the narcissistic fragility encountered in the women seen in our clinical practice. Concerning the first trimester, it is pointed out that this period would be marked by ambivalence, with little elaboration of the ghosts related to pregnancy and maternity.

Through clinical experience, it is found that women sometimes live this trimester in denial, sometimes acting as if they were not pregnant (which could also occur in natural pregnancies). Although the scenario described by Faria cannot be generalized to all cases of egg donation, it is certainly applicable to some cases.

In the second trimester of pregnancy, the woman notices the physiological changes and is sensitive to the psychological ones. Aware of the fetal movements of the baby that grows inside her, a cut is established in the mother-fetus symbiosis. The child's fantasy begins to be generated, the mother realizes that the process is not totally in her control and that the baby will have its own characteristics; these characteristics in the mother's fantasy are the result of the genesis of two distinct babies: the wonderful baby (imaginary baby) and the bad baby, the result of original sin in the Judeo-Christian mentality (Faria, 2005). From the genesis of these two will be built the real child.

This fantasy movement of the baby becomes peculiar in donor fertilization, considering that the genetic information is only half known. The woman cannot relate to a baby whom she does not fantasize about, the need arises to fantasize the origin of the baby: the donor woman. Thus, it ends up assuming two possibilities: that of a wonderful woman or a horrible woman, both influencing and / or compromising the connection with the baby, requiring psychological work to elaborate the fantasies.

According to Faria (2005), it becomes impossible for women to support a baby without a face, there may be an increase in the fantasy of malformation, generating a physical and psychological malaise of the second trimester and a longing for the end. Premature births become understandable, as the expulsion of the baby means the answer to their questions. (Faria, 2005).

Gabriel had been born at 35 weeks, after a major fight between Paulo and Paula. The difficulties in recognizing this baby and feeling him as one's own can bring with it the fantasy of adultery of the partner with the donor, presenting the partner as the biological father, the donor as the biological mother, and the recipient as the one who is only asked to be the mother of the baby of the other.

Paula did not clearly express this fantasy, but it was put into words by Paulo when after the separation of the couple, he reported that now he and his son would be free to look for the donor and Gabriel could finally have a mother and the three of them could start a family.

In oocyte donation, the non-resolution of infertility is very marked, since the child born is the real representation of the woman's disability. The depressive feelings and the difficulty in the relationship with the child show this narcissistic fragility. The issues of self-esteem and the feelings of worthlessness can be compensated by excessive protection of the child, which can hide the real difficulties of the mother in establishing a bond with her child, remembering here, once again, Paula's excessive concern with Gabriel.

Another important aspect to note is the significance of gamete donations, as well as the circulation of this material outside the body. Perelson (2020) talks about the autonomization of gametes. They circulate, are extracted, frozen, manipulated, discarded, marketed, donated, received. He states that the donations and receptions of free gametes create new forms of psychic and social bonds, without considering the symbolic and imaginary place in the construction of affiliation and the construction of parenthood that donors will have. The author tells us about a social bond that is created between donor and recipient.

We could think of a phantom bond between the two, a permanent and sometimes persecutory bond. The donor must mourn her donated eggs, while the recipient must mourn not being the mother of her child. To donors, the child owes his coming into the world and parents owe their exercise of parenting.

Eggs end up being gifts of life. In this regard, Genevieve de Perseval and Pierre Verdier (1994) reflect on what leads people to donate their gametes, pointing to a metapsychology of donation. The biological tissues related to filiation are, for the authors, mythical products, they are metaphors because what is donated is not the egg or semen, but life or something that can create it.

In their opinion, the donation would be linked to the anal phase and would follow the line of the stool-penis-babies equation, being seen as a gift that is offered to someone, like the stool that children offer to those they love, but also to those who at some point they feel hatred or resentment towards, even though these donations seem to function as genitalized donations: donors of anonymous children and recipients of anonymous children (Perseval & Verdier, 1994).

If we refer here to what donors and recipients say, we see that through the donation of these vital substances there is a certain appropriation of the other, as we give him something he did not have. In this appropriation, the idea of domination is present, but also, clearly, the brand. In fact, donors transmit these famous links that we talk about, links that are supposed to have a genetic sense, but also a symbolic one (Perseval & Verdier, 1994).

This symbolic link, filiation, is recognition and knowledge: for the parents, it is the child's place in the narcissistic continuity. Filiation is the recognition of one's own position in the order of generations, recognition that the desire of the parents precedes the existence of the child, which means the registration of the child in the tree of the ancestors, as well as his integration within the law (Bregazzi, 2019).

So, the occult origins may constitute an attack or manipulation of the parents. Symbolic filiation is a continuity that announces a break: one is born into a family to later be born into the family, where the dreamed child is replaced by the real child, especially when there is a need for help to obtain parenthood. This need is experienced as a threat to parental potency.

Another narcissistic wound would be linked to the fact that these parents have to seek, for example, therapeutic help for a child, again facing a disability, creating a family crisis. If the parents deny the difficulties, what is expressed is the difficulty with the intimate filiatory bond (Bregazzi, 2019).

Already in the initial interviews with the mother, it seemed to the analyst that this symbolic place within a family had not been given to Gabriel, but it remained to be seen. In the first session, Gabriel seemed embarrassed but soon started talking about how angry his mother was because he did not know how to write stories and how upset he was about not knowing how to draw because his colleagues knew how to draw very well. He really wanted to learn how to draw, but he couldn't. So he copied drawings and as his mother was very dedicated, she had put the boy in a drawing course. He asked the analyst if she wanted to see his drawings and started drawing animals, all with very strong pencils.

In the following sessions, he continued to try to copy animal drawings, but his outline ended up creating bizarre figures. As the analysis progressed, Gabriel allowed himself to make freer drawings, but they were drawings of loose elements: bombs, toilets, feces that flew through the sheet of paper, along with astronauts and monsters. It was as if Gabriel perceived several of this elements, but could not put them together.

After a few months of analysis, Gabriel began to be interested in games, and in a given session he arrived at the office and proposed to play Clue (in Clue there is a crime, a secret that needs to be unraveled, as well as who committed it and which weapon was used).

G: Now I can almost guess the weapon!
A: Really, that fast?!
G: Yeah, I almost know.

The "almost know" seemed to refer to knowing part of his history, even though he could not connect the elements.

We continued playing and he headed for the cemetery space.

G: It's better to die in the cemetery because then you'll be buried right there.

"Dying in the cemetery" could mean his sense of non-existence in the face of a story of which Gabriel knew only a few pieces, as well as how much he felt invaded by deadly aspects, seeing himself as responsible for the death of the other babies.

When the game was over, Gabriel mentioned:

G: How strange?
A: What's strange?
G: This thing here, the English punch.
A: And why is it strange?
G: Because it's English, it's from somewhere else.
A: There must be a lot of strange things, things from somewhere else in your life that you don't understand.
G: Yeah, there are.

In another session Gabriel talked about his original fantasy: "*I was born of desemination*", creating a neologism because the correct phrase would be: "of insemination".

A: And what is this?
G: I saw it on TV. There was a report in the news and father said that I was born that way.
A: And how was that?

G: It was while I was a liquid.

A: Liquid?

G: I was a liquid and my father's DNA wasn't coming. Then they took me out of my mother's belly, where I was a liquid, and they took my father's DNA and then put me back in my mother's belly.

Gabriel revealed that he clearly knew his story, that is, he carried only his father's DNA, but despite his knowledge, his story needed to be denied and contradicted.

Many gamete donations will be kept secret. Regarding secrets, Mann (2018) points out that they can affect the children's sense of trust in their parents, creating a potential imbalance in their psychic functions and their object relations.

In another session, Gabriel decided to draw the family. He presented a lot of difficulty in drawing, and his fine motor skills were very poor. He picked up the sheet and held it in front of him:

G: I can't draw. I don't know how to draw. I have some magazines at home that teach you how, but I'm getting better. But I can't draw the family, I can't remember everyone's face. I don't have a very good memory, I can't remember anything. I can't remember the day of the week, the order of the months, I can't even remember now. Can't it be a random family?

By saying he couldn't remember his family and asking if he could draw a random family, Gabriel seemed to reveal once again his perception that he didn't belong, revealing the strangeness he felt, while at the same time taking responsibility for his difficulties: his memory problems. Bayo-Borrás (2020) questions what would be the difference in the neurotic family novel in children born by gamete donation.

In what was described by Freud ([1909] 1996), there is information about the origin that was hidden and that corresponds to a much better version. In children born by gamete donation, if they live the experience that something has been hidden, there is a lie and a pretense about information vital for the constitution of their identity. The children of donors are subjected to uncertainties about their identity and that of their unknown parents and are not sure if they can trust their mothers and fathers, as they suspect their silences, the incomplete stories told, and the efforts to find physical similarities.

For Bayo-Borràs (2020), one of the inevitable problems is the "revelation" of the origin. Parents tend to keep techno-reproductive procedures muted and hidden even from close family and friends, as well as their own children. Thus, this aspect, so significant for the identity of each person, becomes a great "state" secret.

She also questions what the effects might be on children's subjectivity and states that they will receive the message that asking and wanting to know can lead to dangerous places, and that knowing about themselves is uncomfortable for their parents. Another frequently observed consequence is difficulties in school learning. The cognitive functions of thinking for oneself can also be affected, establishing collusion with the parents' unconscious.

Gabriel could not ask, he could not write stories, he could not have curiosity. He needed to take full responsibility for his difficulties and with that, he needed to prove himself perfect, to perhaps give a minimum of satisfaction to his mother.

G: I can't draw. I know, I'm going to draw something that I've already been able to draw perfectly: a flamingo. Do you know flamingos?
A: I do.
G: They're pink and they're all the same. I tried to draw people, but I wasted a lot of paper. Do you know that drawing is like writing?

For Kupfer (1989), what is at stake for the child is the need, first of all, to know his place in the world, a sexual place, where the question "where do we come from and where do we go?", which is related to the parents, expresses the desire to know what the parents expect from the child, what the parents' desire is concerning the child. For the author, "Where did we come from" is equivalent to "What is my origin in relation to your desire?", "why did you put me in the world?", "to meet what expectations?", "so that I become what I am?" (where are we heading?).

We are in the field of the Oedipus Complex or an Oedipus Frankenstein (Bayo-Borràs, 2020), so called due to the nature of the bonds created with the different characters involved, as well as the articulation of scientific and individual desires, which can interfere with the subjectivity of those involved.

In another session, he once again revealed his perceptions and the need to attack them:

G: I always give explanations. I don't like injustice, so I always explain and it usually works.
A: What kind of injustice?
G: Like lying too. I can't think of any. The things I say are because of my IQ, so I forget.
A: I think you're quite intelligent and then you become aware of the things that happen in your life and then you try to forget them.
G: I don't have a good memory.

Gabriel's analysis continued for two years, with many difficulties in helping him integrate these aspects within himself, coupled with the mother's difficulties in understanding that her desires and fantasies directly affected the boy's development; until it was interrupted by Paula's change of job.

Final considerations

The case introduces us to the theme of motherhood (parenting) and the arrival of children with the help of assisted reproduction techniques. Gabriel was born by egg donation and this was a family secret. This fact allows us to think about how this experience is inscribed within a particular bond for each couple, that is, how these experiences are processed in each individual, at the psychic level.

In the first interview, the mother already appears alone, marking the absence of Gabriel's father. During the consultation, the father's voice is not heard, even when invited. The mother reports that he has conduct problems, she does not say what they are, and he is an absent father. Later on, we will understand that the so-called "conduct issues" meet very unrealistic fantasies and desires: finding the donor and forming a family with her.

The parents are in the process of divorce, which signals a history that is breaking. Is that also why Gabriel can't write stories? How can one talk about a broken bond where it's not really known when it actually broke or if it was ever a loving bond capable of sustaining a family?

In the first interviews, almost like a confession, Paula reveals that Gabriel is not her son. We are in the field of differences between genitor and father, and genitor and mother. The female genitor is the one who donates the gametes but renounces subjectivity and the exercise of parenthood; the mother is the one who carries out the parental project, exercising the functions of support (maternal function).

Gabriel has his father's genes, but this does not seem to drive Paulo to exercise the paternal function. On the other hand, he does not have his mother's genetics and she is not able to fully exercise her maternal function when she says "he is not my son". She solves this by saying: "João is like me, while Gabriel is like his father".

She divides her children, showing that she is not linked to Gabriel. He doesn't belong to her. One for each of you. Here we have another unconstituted bond. There is no symbolic adoption.

The maintenance of the secret is directly linked to the narcissistic wound experienced by Paula, in the face of infertility and early menopause, so she is enraged when her husband decides to tell Gabriel about his origin. Nothing can change, you need to keep everything as it is, denying the infertility and Gabriel's origin. Secrets, family romance, breaking ties. Gabriel is a detective in his own life and claims to know everything. Does he know his origin? His history? Does he know it and can't write it down? Does he know it and can't tell it?

On the other hand, will he have enough psychic resources to search for his origins and find out what happened to his parents? How will he experience the fantasy of his family romance? But like Oedipus, death appears in the patient's association. Dying in the cemetery, already staying there. I'm already dead. Can Gabriel leave the cemetery? Does he have a life outside?

Death fantasies pervade Gabriel all the time. Staying in the cemetery is also staying with the other dead embryos. Why would he be the only survivor? What would have happened to the others? In the mourning that is done, the dead are buried. Was there a process of elaboration for these losses?

Following the session, he talks about the strangeness in front of the English punch. It's weird because it's from somewhere else. There is a mark that says where it comes from, there is a new reference to the origin and he states: "I was born by desemination", in a condensation of the word insemination. Dissemination, to disseminate, to spread over many parts. Gabriel is a scattered child? Apart? Like the different elements he draws. He continues talking about his theories as to the origin, stating that he was liquid and that they placed him in his mother's belly, which did not belong to him. How does one psychically represent the idea of being taken, mixed, and placed in the mother's belly?

When asked about who his family is, he also does not include his father, he says he does not know how to draw, he needs to copy, and he lacks models to continue being or to constitute himself. Drawing is like writing, he tells us that both functions are compromised, he cannot express himself if he does not know who he is, and he calls forth the flamingos, which are all the same.

Although assisted reproduction techniques have existed for more than 40 years and currently happen on a large scale, we are still unaware of the complex effects that their use generate on the individuals involved (donors, parents, and children). It is certain, however, that in Gabriel his genetic origin, distinct from the mother, was the driving force for the difficulties in the mother-child bond, present from the beginning of his history, increasing secrets and lies that were at the service of "saving" maternal narcissism, already overthrown. The impossibility of recognizing Gabriel as a son, his history, means that the boy has to attack his perceptions all the time, because of the violent reality that is imposed on him. We have a great risk to the psychic life of Gabriel, who does not find shelter in a third organizing and structuring function, but on the contrary, finds himself facing a delusional father who also attacks reality.

The lack of recognition of the symbolic filiation resulted in a history of maladjustments between Gabriel and his mother, allied to the paternal difficulties of assuming a position of third function, which also seem to have caused maladjustments between Gabriel and his father. A few months of analysis were necessary for him to be able to begin to express his perceptions and anxiety, but these were always attacked, as there was a need to keep a secret. Narcissistic aspects of the parents predominated to the detriment of Gabriel's recognition of his otherness.

Gabriel knows his story, he really needs to put it in order, but for that he needs parents who are good enough to help him tell it, to write it down. What is certain is that we still have to think about the psychic consequences that assisted reproduction technologies create in the subjects involved with them.

References

Badinter, E. (1980). *Um amor conquistado: O mito do amor materno*. Editora Nova Fronteira.

Bayo-Borrás, R. (2020). En busca del parentesco desconocido. Reproducción Humana Asistida, Bioética y Psicoanálisis. *Revista Digital de Psicoterapia Psicoanalítica*, 9: 1–18.

Bregazzi, C. (2019). Procesos de filiación "intervenidos" ¿Hay lugar para el pensamiento, la conjetura, la intimidad? *Controversias en Psicoanálisis de Niños y Adolescentes*, 24: 89–99.

Faria, C. (2005). Amor de mães: A experiência gravídica e parentalidade na fertilização com óvulos de doador. In I. Leal (Ed.). *Psicologia da gravidez e da parentalidade* (pp. 145–157). Fim de Século.

Fiorini, L. (2001). *Lo femenino y el pensamento complejo*. Lugar Editorial.

Freud, S. ([1909] 1996). *Romances familiares*. In S. Freud, *Edição Standard Brasileira das Obras Psicológicas Completas de Sigmund Freud, volume IX* (pp. 189–202). Imago.

Kupfer, M. C. N. (1989). *Psicanálise do diagnóstico estrutural*. Casa do Psicólogo.

Mann, M. (2018). *Psychoanalytic aspects of assisted reproductive technology*. Routledge.

Perelson, S. (2020). Sobre as práticas de dons de ovócitos no Brasil e na França: Dom, mercado, ciência. In L. Fulgencio, D. Kupermann, E. L. Cunha, & J. Birman (Eds.). *Amar a si mesmo e amar o outro* (pp. 162–184). Zagodoni.

Perseval, G., & Verdier, P. (1994). *Enfant de personne*. Odille Jacob.

Tubert, S. (1996). Psicoanálisis, feminismo, postmodernismo. In M. Burín & E. Dio-Bleichmar (Eds.). *Género, Psicoanálisis, subjetividad*. Paidós.

Chapter 11

Motherhood without pregnancy
Surrogacy, a challenge for femininity and maternal preoccupation

Christine Anzieu-Premmereur

Introduction

Assisted reproductive technology helps to achieve parenthood in ways so that pregnancy can now be undertaken by a surrogate who gets paid for getting the fertilized egg after hormonal stimulation and carrying the pregnancy, while renouncing raising the child. Parents wish to be in control of a difficult process when choosing egg, sperm or surrogate for the baby they have dreamed about and will "adopt" as a familiar newborn, or as a foreign one. There is such a huge hope to have a baby and to be a parent! But this is different from classical adoption, when parents who have had to mourn their own reproductive capabilities, choose to adopt and raise a baby that has already been conceived by biological parents.

Finding a woman willing to carry a pregnancy amongst family or friends, or hiring one for money, is a specific process that allows for adopting a baby created with some genetic material from the intended parents and following the pregnancy in the surrogate. This allows for overcoming infertility or inability to bear a pregnancy, as in the case of some mothers who already suffered medical or mental issues during a previous pregnancy. This chapter will explore how this very specific kind of mothering can foster or alienate the capacity for maternal preoccupation.

The Winnicottian notion of primary maternal preoccupation ([1956] 1975) we are alluding to, states that, because of a mother's intense identification with her infant and the unconscious memories of having been cared for, activated by the presence of her child, the mother gradually develops a state of heightened sensitivity, almost an illness. In this model, the infant and mother are almost merged.

Any newborn – whatever the method of conception – always has to be "adopted" to become familiar, similar, part of the family. The postpartum period is an especially sensitive time that makes a new mother able to regress, to identify with the primitive needs and emotions of the newborn, to make familiar this "new stranger in the home", as Anne Bouchard-Godard (1993) wrote. The puerperal hormonal changes are the cause of some intense

DOI: 10.4324/9781032693446-11

emotional reactions that help or interfere with the mother's adjusting to her new identity and role, and it has been observed that some adopting mothers have strong hormonal reactions to the presence of the new baby.

The question of the ability to love and to identify with the new foreign baby is not specific to adopting mothers. Any woman has to make that move. Pregnancy helps that process, since the body's changes and the time passing transform the woman's fantasmatic representations of herself as a mother and of the new baby.

When motherhood happens without pregnancy, there was previously a long journey towards parenthood, and that painful time with a lot of hope has also been a time for representing and imagining. The same issues regarding intense ambivalence towards the baby we can find in adopting mothers, we can also find in anxious new mothers, and that ambivalence can interfere with the necessary regression to infantile sexuality, when strong defences lead to the inability to touch the infant or when the prevalent narcissistic cathexis towards the child makes that precious baby interesting only as a precocious preforming child. Piera Aulagnier (1975) has stressed the difference between the desire for pregnancy and motherhood, but without any desire for a real child, there is no space for a separated new life, for a baby with a body and vital and attachment needs.

Complex ambivalent desires

Guilt feelings towards her own parents and the surrogate can result in submission to all the child's demands without limit, in a need for expiation, while at the same time projecting onto the infant a grandiosity associated with all the narcissistic wishes that are part of this very controlled creation of a baby.

Oedipus was an adopted child who dramatically discovered his two kinds of filiation, genetic and adoptive. He learned how adoption was associated with essential issues, not only incest prohibition, but also how biological filiation helps for narcissistic reassurance. This family story is always a new reality for mothers who face sterility, with the risk of loving their children too intensely, without symbolic limits.

Becoming a mother activates an intrapsychic reorganization. Motherhood without pregnancy can be for a daughter a privileged occasion to continue her primitive relationship with her mother. Giving birth can be for some pregnant women an experience of traumatic separation, while for others having a baby allows for regressing at being again in an archaic relationship with a maternal figure (Anzieu-Premmereur, 2011).

Mostly unconscious, the capacity to hold in mind another person and to be devoted to his bodily as well as psychological needs is part of mothering. But this capacity is also an essential component of creativity in men and women, whether they are parents or not, making them able to care for others and develop a subtle adjustment to them.

The mother's unconscious ability to be attentive, to hold her child in her mind and with her body, attuned to his/her feelings and needs, able to deal with his/her disorganized and sometimes unbearable emotions, plus her love and her identification with the child, her attachment and her tenderness, fosters the development of the child's felt experience as continuous, consistent, predicable, and as owned by the child, as "mine".

This maternal function gives the child an envelope for his/her own functioning that can be contained and then felt as a personal experience. The infant's self, or premature ego, internalizes this maternal capacity.

The consequences of this maternal capacity not only impact the quality of the boundaries of the ego and the solidity of healthy narcissism, but also affect the internalization of this capacity. Some of us are better able to be attuned to others and to use our own mind to hold the minds of others. This applies of course to psychoanalysts and their ability to engage in transference-countertransference interchange.

Donald Winnicott ([1956] 1975) has beautifully described this very special sensitivity in the new mother that allows her to be fully attentive to the baby's immaturity and dependence. By identifying herself to the baby, the mother achieves a very powerful sense of what the baby needs; she knows what the infant feels and is able to provide almost exactly what he needs. This is a live adaptation to the infant's needs. And this process is supposed to end when the baby needs to separate. The primary maternal preoccupation is a specific state of mind, close to a personality split but without becoming schizoid, in which most mothers enter while giving birth. Adoptive mothers can also get this special sensitivity to be tender and attuned to their baby.

Primary maternal preoccupation presupposes both a bodily and an affective state in the woman as mother, but this maternal ability is a challenge for the woman's narcissism. If she has had trouble identifying with her own mother, if she is still dreaming of a merger with an archaic mother, or if her mind is full of incestuous fantasies, she will be vulnerable. In fact, some women are not able to become preoccupied with their own infant to the exclusion of other interests in this way. So these women may feel they have to make up for it later, until the time has passed and the deadline to get pregnant creates the urge to find a solution at any price.

The specificity of the woman as woman and not only as mother is often excluded from observations of motherhood. Maternal function at the centre of psychoanalytic attention and the concern for the infant's mental health tend to reduce the woman to her role as mother. After thinking about the development of a girl's femininity and how it relates to her ability to become a mother, this chapter will show the specificity of parental issues when having a baby through a surrogate: starting with the role of identification in building a feminine identity and describing the genetic continuity between early sexual phases in childhood and adolescence, the adventure of motherhood develops with the trials and vicissitudes of the feminine development.

Femininity and identifications

Feminine and maternal identification play a very important role in building the human being's psychic development. Both the identification to the mother as a woman, and the identification to the mother as a mother, are the roots of feminine narcissism. The girl identifies with both the archaic mother figure and the Oedipal mother image: the mother's psychic bisexuality is at the origin of the female identity of the daughter.

Florence Guignard (2002) wrote about primary femininity as being related to the first object loss during weaning. Greed for the mother's body and excitement of the precocious sexual drives are both intense. This is the time when an object other than the self is first recognized, when the process of introjection is organized and reinforced. Depending on the mother's ability for "maternal *rêverie*", as Bion (1962) wrote, the introjective process is also related to the beginning of the depressive position, allowing for the opportunity to deal with mourning and guilt.

A second post-Oedipal phase contributes with another layer of femininity. The ambivalence towards the pre-Oedipal mother is resolved by the girl's later adolescent identification with the maternal function. Nonetheless, the girl doesn't abandon her pre-Oedipal attachment to her mother, and this fluidity between infantile attachments and adult personality is easy to observe during pregnancy.

Internalization of conflict and identification with the mother are the early steps in formation of the superego: we see the girl's efforts to resolve conflicting feelings of love and hate towards her mother. This internalization implies idealization of the mother and of her directives, and harsh introjects are turned against the self at any hint of libidinal or aggressive impulse. The wish for a sense of closeness with the idealized mother and the fear of losing her love are central motivators in the development of the female superego, just as issues of gender, narcissism and self-esteem are closely bound with superego development. A confident sense of femininity and the wish to assume a feminine gender role, and eventually the wish to take the mother's place in relation to the father, are dependent on the girl's having made selective identifications with the idealized mother.

If the girl is able to deal successfully with the challenge and the frustration, compromise and internal modification become easier. She is then able to maintain greater interpersonal and intrapsychic harmony and is more easily able to retain an inner sense of the mother as a constant libidinal object. When anxiety over loss of the mother's love becomes overwhelming, the girl's evaluation of her femininity may be compromised; she may fail to find pleasure in shared female gender-role activities and instead an intense sadomasochistic relationship with the mother ensues (Benedek, 1959).

During this phase, the father can significantly help the girl in building a valued sense of her own femininity by helping her resolve rapprochement ambivalence and by encouraging her to identify with her mother. New identifications with a female gender role pave the way for triadic object relations. The girl's fantasy is now to play the role of the mother towards the father. Such wishes interfere with concurrent wishes for mother's love, so that previous object-related wishes and conflicts become reorganized with triadic object relations. Envy, jealousy and anger towards each parent, fear of loss of love, low self-esteem and guilt accompany these fantasies.

Many variations of conflict are possible for the girl, while she strives to satisfy libidinal and aggressive urges and simultaneously gains a measure of impulse control to meet the standards of the emergent superego. She is also attempting to maintain her mother's love in face of the desire to compete with her for the father's affection. At the same time, she is trying to consolidate a narcissistically valued sense of femininity. She is striving to maintain self-esteem in the face of ungratified wishful fantasies. The nature of the strong tie to the mother and the girl's difficulty in moving beyond it are central to achieving triadic relations. In fact, the infantile neurosis has roots in dyadic, pre-Oedipal object relations.

Organizers of motherhood and maternal preoccupation

A new mother will have to reorganize her identifications, replaying her infantile desires. She will identify, in an intense projective activity, her infant with her own past representations, in a close relation to her infantile narcissism delegated into the infant.

The parental feelings of loss associated with infertility can unconsciously engage the child in a fantasmatic transformation of those experiences, with intense wishes to have the child fully protected against any pain of frustration or loss. The observation of negative reactions in infants towards their mothers, avoiding touching and looking at them, has shown the pathological consequences of lack of pleasure and libidinal cathexis.

The libidinal and aggressive drives that animate the projective identification towards the child are in direct relation to the quality of elaboration of the parents' mourning process. Palacio Espasa (2004) has developed the idea that becoming a parent confronts oneself with a "developmental process of mourning". The young adult must cede the place she had occupied before with her parents to the new baby. As well, the presence of the infant forces her to assume the role of the parent.

The mother's discovery of the newborn's absolute dependence may have a traumatic impact on her and make it almost impossible to carry out the psychic transformation underlying the access to parenthood. The new mother has to deal again with the primary relation to the object. Her own ability to protect her baby is formed from her experience of having been dependent on her mother. Bowlby (1969) explained how the first experience of dependency builds the roots for the future independence: when the child has been able to keep an internal image of the mother, he can separate from her.

So the mothers who have experienced a disturbed primary relationship with their own mothers will be confronted with difficulty in mothering. The normal ambivalence towards the baby brings back the memory of the negative feelings towards her own mother, or the reality of the baby can stir up incestuous fantasies and the fear associated with it. When the new mother doesn't have the protection of an infantile, well-structured neurosis that allows a psychic working-through of the archaic fantasies, she will be at risk of a paranoid crisis: her ego defences will be overwhelmed. Her fears concerning her own integrity and identity will be projected onto the infant.

If a mother, adopting or not, has suffered from previous loss or narcissistic wounding without being able to recover, she will be overwhelmed with guilt and aggression. The newborn is not the same as the baby she has had in her dreams since she was a little girl, nor a narcissistic duplicate of herself. The postpartum blues could be a temporary crisis that allows the mother to identify with the helpless infant, or it could be the start of a depressive state that lasts, with feelings of emptiness, uselessness and all the consequences of a disturbed attachment.

The desire for a child is always a complex ambivalent wish. The impossibility of having a child naturally may transform this desire into a need. A conflicted urge towards parenthood can transform the desire into an obligation.

In assisted reproduction, future parents are involved into such a physical, psychological and emotional participation, and their intense desire might saturate everything, body and mind (Nayar-Akhtar, 2014). Sexual pleasure, spontaneity and intimacy are replaced by suffering. The primal scene is the place of origin for each one of us. When the plan to have a child is separated from the sexual act, what fantasies does this stimulate?

Biotechnologies introduce an artificial element to overcome the limits posed by nature and this alien element poses a challenge for some. A biological part of another human being, or a woman carrying the fetus, strangers involved in the creation of the baby can be experienced as interfering or as supports that can be integrated into the family. The role of the medical intervention can be experienced as taking the central role and eliminating the couple and/or the woman as the center of parenthood. The child's origin may remain an open issue in the child as in the parents, and establish itself as a "family secret" (Marion, 2017). The secret triggers guilt, shame and the difficulty of integrating the medical interventions. This leaves the child facing the unsaid about his origin and the force of denial.

Like in infantile sexual theories, the parents' sexuality has been denied by the medical intervention. We may wonder if the representation of the original scene of procreation is no longer fundamental. If so, which fantasies are then at play? Do they integrate the roles of pleasure and sexuality?

Whatever these combinations, in the majority of cases we will find a good-enough mix of life and death sexual drives, of ethical ability and of vital narcissism in the parents' psyche, even though proper genital sexuality has been either partially or completely excluded from procreation. This good-enough mix lies at the basis of a good-enough child development for what concerns the unavoidable impact of the parental environment upon the child's psychic formation. In fact, the goal of the analytic and psychotherapeutic interventions is to achieve this good-enough mixing (Chétrit-Vatine, 2012).

Surrogate mothers can be a friend or family member ready to help; while they are often women who need money, some are very motivated by the wish to give a baby to another mother. The conflicts around guilt and debt that are already at stake in any motherhood – the debt of life towards their own mothers that new mothers experience, and that make some give the baby to their parents –, will play an important role in the capability for the intended mother to feel legitimate. This differs from regular adoption when the parents have chosen the surrogate and made a contract with her to go through IVF to carry their own biological parts. Some feminist authors have developed the argument of legalization of surrogacy to avoid exploitation and to create a different society where gestational assistance would be altruistic and lead to a "polymaternal" parenting, erasing social differences. The surrogate would be a part of the child's life, making parents less stressed by the demands of the baby (Lewis, 2019).

Parental projections

Some parents seem to keep an identity as sterile parents towards a child that is always the proof of their infertility (Ansermet, Meijia Quijano & Germond, 2006). Filiation has always been more a symbolic function than a biological process. Now that sperm, eggs, even embryos can be exchanged, sold, exposed on the Internet, now that uterus can be rented, the business is faster than the law system in most countries. Children with three different origins – sperm, egg and uterus – all distinct from their parents, are facing a symbolic system that has to be created. Thinking of reproduction outside of sexuality, but inside a symbolic frame of filiation, is a complex process and is a new source of anxiety, mostly to the medical and psychotherapeutic community.

New couples face the challenge to re-evaluate their own identity as parents, which is very different from their experience during their own childhood. The infantile omnipotent wish for a baby, stimulated when biology doesn't allow it, can organize in some vulnerable patients a defence as denial of sterility. This doesn't allow for a mourning process and the transformation of the trauma. "Where does my baby come from?" remains a constant question.

After the birth of the child, the complexity of the meeting with the real child, the projections of the narcissistic issues regarding his/her origins, can put the mother-infant dyad at risk. We have to think about the baby's psychic development in this specific context. The parent's own pregenital and Oedipal history and cathexis will play a fundamental role in the transmission of meaning to the child (Ehrensaft, 2008). The mutual identification between mother and infant is under the mother's own infantile unconscious representation of being female. This specific interaction helps the mother's cathexis of her capacity to contain babies.

The uterus can be experienced as a sexual organ or as a silent part of the body, assimilated to the digestive system in an anal investment. The capacity for representation of the internal organs is here at stake. Sometimes one's uterus is not differentiated from a representation of the mother's one. For some, this leads to a repetition of infantile issues, which could eventually play a role in the cathexis of the baby after the birth, and the relationship with a baby girl (Guignard, 2002).

Some of those new mothers coming for consultation with their infant are dealing with despair at not being able to love their newborn, or believing their child couldn't attach to them. Some have dissociated themselves from any feeling and sensation, functioning in a concrete mechanical behaviour, like in the "blank depression" described by André Green (1993). They couldn't find any pleasure in the bodily contact with the child. The analyst then has to label their negative feelings as sadness and anger, which are sometimes projected into the baby.

The trauma of the past sterility, the miscarriages, IVF, medical treatments and anxiety over the pregnancy has made them extremely sensitive to any judgment about their capability for mothering a child. We may observe how becoming a parent signifies confronting a developmental process of mourning for the future parent (Palacio Espasa, 2004), who must cede the place he had occupied as his parents' child. The presence of the infant makes the couple assume the role of the parent in an interactive dynamic between identification with the child and libidinal and aggressive drives.

Compared with the disarray of pregnant women who had a traumatic birth and the accompanying sense of helplessness and narcissistic trauma, the mother who receives a newborn from a surrogate, even if she identifies with the woman giving birth, has no changes in her body. She may have missed pregnancy, and the intense bodily preparation for caring for an infant body, but she has not suffered from what some women during postpartum go through, which can also interfere with the ability to love the child.

Again, what of the maternal preoccupation in the adoptive mother without the hormonal changes and the nine months of representation of the creation of a child? Most women, and parents, who have chosen egg donor, sperm donor and surrogate, create plenty of representations of the future child, figurations that are associated with their own transgenerational fantasies.

For instance, the mother of a baby boy created by surrogacy had the fantasy of a mental illness in the surrogate that had made the infant sleepless. A few sessions helped the baby to fall asleep, and the parents discovered that their fantasy was associated with the frightening maternal figure of the maternal grandmother being angry with the omnipotent medical creation of the boy.

The painful absence of maternal preoccupation will be at the centre of the case of a young woman who suffered severe postpartum depression and abandoned her baby girl for a period of time.

Susan, a mother who abandoned her child after a surrogate pregnancy

I met with Susan after she had a baby through a surrogate mother impregnated with Susan's egg and her husband's sperm, due to a medical condition. A few months after the birth, she had abandoned the baby girl to the father. When I met her, she was in the process of recovering from a severe depression and "adopting her daughter".

She reported that during her teenage years, she had dreamed of having a baby she would keep with her forever. But she discovered she had an anatomic issue in her uterus that made her unable to maintain a pregnancy. She was eager to do whatever worked, had her eggs frozen with the husband's sperm and found a surrogate among their relatives. When her daughter Anna was born, looking at her for the first time, she thought: "You, you'll have to manage on your own". She felt love, but no bond.

Susan consulted with me about Anna when she was four-years-old and was running away from her. Her little girl ran away every day, in the garden, in the playground, in the street in the middle of traffic. Susan didn't know what to do since she froze up and could only look silently at Anna who ignored her. Talking to me, she began to be aware how dangerous the situation was. She remembered what she had said to the babysitter: "I wouldn't be upset with you if something terrible happened to my daughter". She then realized it was a death wish.

I met with Anna. She was playing out an Oedipal scenario with dolls. I interpreted her guilt and the fear that I would punish her because she ran away from her mother. She said her mother never punished her, even when she was mean!

I recommended psychotherapy for Susan; she agreed. She said she was full of guilt, thinking she was the cause of her daughter's behavior. She could let Anna disappear and she realized that other parents wouldn't behave like her, since "there was a bond between them and their children"; a bond she didn't feel. Anna was surprised, listening to her mother. I remembered her the guilt she reported a few minutes before, and I asked her if she was running away because she was angry. "Yes", she said, "because my mom was so sick". Then Susan explained she had been so depressed, she felt so empty and desperate that she was unable to contain her child's feelings, to meet her needs. She decided to leave home for a year. Anna had stayed with the father, waiting for her mother to return. She had been abandoned.

When Susan recovered from the depression she started to meet with her daughter but she was disappointed. It was difficult for her to spend a whole day with Anna since she didn't know how to set up limits. Anna started to scream in the street, to be upset, and then to run away.

As soon as we started psychotherapy, Susan began to feel a separation anxiety she didn't know she had experienced before. She realized she hadn't felt the bond that a mother usually feels. Slowly, working with me on her paradoxical relationship with her grandmother, who had raised her while her own mother wasn't available, she became aware of the repetition of abandonments. She experienced a rage towards the surrogate, a half-sister of her father, a nurse always devoted to others. Between fusion and hatred, she started to feel a link between her and her daughter. She reported having the fantasy that the running child was looking for the surrogate mother as the only place to be secure. Full of thoughts for her child during the night, she was sad to be lonely. She said, "I miss an attachment". Then she recovered a kind of maternal preoccupation, thinking of her daughter day and night.

Susan decided to ask for a divorce and to fight to have custody of Anna. After a very painful trial, she gained the right to have her daughter living with her. She became able to set limits and to tell her young daughter she had feared losing her. She told her she loved her and would never leave her alone again. Keeping Anna close to her body and always present in her mind, she prevented the girl's running away.

During the first year of the therapy, she recovered a better narcissistic foundation. In a very positive transference towards me, she used me as a mirror reflecting her conflicts, without being judged by me. Her guilt lessened. She could then face her own ambivalence towards her mother, as towards her child.... And towards me: having to pay me after missing a session made her overwhelmed with anger. She said that she was the one who suffered from my absence when she didn't come to a session, but it was her who had to give me something, with the risk of feeling totally empty. In the transference, I was a sadistic superego as she fantasized her own mother had been. Working on her rage, her difficulty with feeling controlled, we touched the roots of her feelings of melancholy: her avidity and her guilt towards her mother. She remembered how she had been clutching onto her mother, always frustrated, in a mix of love, anger, hatred and despair. "It had been a negative bond," she said: glued to her cold mother, afraid of losing her, full of negative feelings and guilt. Remembering her childhood, thinking about her parents having a hard time with their own children, she understood the link with the pathological grandparents, therefore Susan finally stopped complaining. She then became more creative, successful in her work, raising a girl who maintained an ambivalent love for her mother.

Libidinization of the body is essential to protect the very young baby against the consequences of traumatic experiences that lead to anxiety, accumulation of aggression, and attacks associated with self-destructiveness (Anzieu-Premmereur & Cornillot, 2003). If we think that autoeroticism leads to the capability for sexual satisfaction linked with representations, then a baby avoiding contact with the mother and lacking self-pleasurable activities is at risk for being fully dependent on the presence of another person or an external object for calming, satisfaction and pleasure, and to addiction, as a complement for its defect of representations of love objects.

The lack of bodily intimacy with the mother, of skin contact, leaves the infant without skin ego protection against intrusion (Anzieu, [1985] 2016). The mother's skin and body are to be used as a shield against intrusive or excessive stimuli. The baby's introjection of this protective capacity is a source of security and sense of self. The failure of this function can create an early trauma and causes primitive defences. Selma Fraiberg ([1980] 2007) reported her observations of avoidant babies who never turn to their mother and scream in huge distress when needy; she also described those who will manage extreme immobilization when the mother is not a source of protection, using "freezing" as the only way to have the body out of feeling.

To conclude

The absence of maternal preoccupation in Susan for her daughter resulted from a long story of misattunements between her and her own mother and from the narcissistic quality of her relationship with the child's father. It took many months of painful sessions for her to get a representation of the surrogate as a woman carrying the baby, and to slowly differentiate herself from her.

There is a discussion on motherhood without pregnancy about the level of narcissistic investment in the future child. Is this long journey across disappointment, grief and complex choices a source of triumph or of feelings of vulnerability and envy?

Depression may be used as a tool for change, and identification with parental figures will play their role in the shaping of the cathexis towards the new baby. Nine months of pregnancy and the dramatic moment of birth help to make a newborn part of a symbiotic bodily system. Without the hormonal and sensorial experience of the body's changes and the associated daydreaming transformations, the process of entering motherhood will be different.

For some, missing those modifications in the feminine body will be experienced as a loss. For others, their identification with a mother figure facilitates representations of bodily changes in motherhood as imaginary and psychosomatic experiences. Whatever the way to become a mother, a woman deals with her own maternal and paternal figures and idealizations. From there, she can get the libidinal energy to welcome the infant. Falling in love is one of the most exciting and intense parts of mothering an infant. Such a drive activity reorganizes the woman's object relations and bisexuality. This extraordinary experience is fully associated with depressive feelings that make room for a new mental organization and identification with the infantile primitive activity of the baby.

The maternal is not only empathy, the mother opposes the child's refusal, opens him/her to the world, offers to act out his/her curiosity. The mother speaks, names everything, she supports language.

There is a traumatic risk in medical interventions concerning reproduction. It's important for psychoanalysts to be aware of the role of preventive interventions, and to make gynecologists and paediatricians aware of the signs of lack of libidinal investment in the pregnancy, as in the baby. Most of the suffering in those cases is quite silent but will have a strong impact on the child's development. Psychoanalytic interventions can help the parents work through their unconscious representations of the origins of the child that may interfere with the infant's own needs.

References

Ansermet, F., Meijia Quijano, C. & Germond, M. (2006). *Parentalité stérile et procréation médicalement assistée*. ERES.

Anzieu, D. ([1985] 2016). *The skin ego*. Karnac.

Anzieu-Premmereur, C. (2011). Fondements maternels de la vie psychique. *Revue française de psychanalyse*, 75: 1449–1488. DOI:10.3917/rfp.755.1449

Anzieu-Premmereur, C. & Cornillot, M. (2003). *Pratiques psychanalytiques avec les bébés*. Dunod.

Aulagnier P. (1975), *La violence de l'interprétation. Du pictogramme à l'énoncé*. Presses Universitaires de France.

Benedek, T. (1959). Parenthood as a developmental phase. *Journal of the American Psychoanalytic Association*, 7: 389–417.

Bion, W. (1962). *Learning from experience*. Basic Books.

Bowlby J. (1969). *L'Attachement*. Presses Universitaires de France.

Bouchard-Godard, A. (1993). Un étranger à demeure. *Devenir*, 5: 43 – 60.

Chétrit-Vatine, V. (2012). *The ethical seduction of the analytic situation; The feminine-maternal origins of responsibility for the other*. Karnac.

Ehrensaft, D. (2008) When baby makes three or four or more. *The Psychoanalytic Study of the Child*, 63: 3–23. DOI: 10.1080/00797308.2008.11800797

Fraiberg S. ([1980] 2007). *Fantômes dans la chambre d'enfants*. Presses Universitaires de France.

Green, A. (1993). The dead mother. *Psyche*, 47: 205–240.

Guignard, F. (2002). *Mère et fille. Entre partage et clivage*. InPress.

Lewis, S. (2019) *Full surrogacy now*. Verso.

Marion, P. (2017). *Il disagio del desiderio. Sessualità e procreazione al tempo delle biotecnologie*. Donzelli Editore.

Nayar-Akhtar, M. (2014). Infertility, trauma, and assisted reproductive technology: Psychoanalytic perspectives. in M. Mann (Ed.), *Psychoanalytic aspects of assisted reproductive technology* (pp. 77–98). Karnac.

Palacio Espasa, F. (2004). Parent-Infant psychotherapy, the transition to parenthood and parental narcissism: Implications for treatment. *Journal of Child Psychotherapy*, 30: 155–171. DOI:10.1080/0075417041000173477

Winnicott D. ([1956] 1975) Primary maternal preoccupation. In *Through paediatrics to psycho-analysis* (pp. 300–305). Basic Books.

Chapter 12

Surrogacy at the origins of the construction of a family

Katy Bogliatto

Introduction

Families formed through surrogacy are nowadays more present in our societies, while nevertheless being a complex technological path of conception for a
child. It is a long process, in which a child can have up to five adults at the
origin of his/her life: the two intended parents – or one in the case of mono-
parental family –, the surrogate carrier (when the woman is also the egg donor)
or the gestational carrier (when the woman has no genetic link), the egg donor,
the sperm donor, or via embryo donation which can be anonymous or known
according to the legal frame of the country.

The common ground between these new family constellations is that they all
need help from ART (assisted reproduction technology), that is, not only a
recourse to a medicalized third-party space, but also to a third-party 'birth-
other' (Ehrensaft, 2000, 2005, 2008). It's a long path, challenging and full of
obstacles, putting to the test everyone involved in the process and requiring for
the parents' specific psychological defenses, strategies, and narratives to accommodate the presence of a 'birth other' in their children's origins. The same
applies for children, who need to process some more specific tasks linked to
their birth-other origins (Ehrensaft, 2008) during their development. This is a
complex challenge that comes on top of the psychic processes of subjectivation
in their individual development, as they negotiate the tasks of attachment,
individuation, and identity in the context of the version of the birth story told
by the parents, in which the infant will construct his own subjective representation of his origin and family history.

Some groundings about surrogacy

Surrogacy raises many questions and controversies that are more preeminent
depending on the part of the world one is looking at it. Nevertheless, one cannot homogenize in a simplistic view such a complex topic. One could say there
are 'different practices of surrogacy', each one of them raising specific

DOI: 10.4324/9781032693446-12

questions linked to legal, economic, ethical, technological, and societal factors characterizing the country or region where the practice takes place, and the country where the intended parents and surrogate or gestational woman live.

Some examples are the economic issue, which, with the financial compensation for the gestational/surrogate woman, raises questions such as the payment for the use of her body and for the result: the child; it also questions the motivations the gestational woman has to embark in a procedure that challenges her body and her internal psychic world, her family environment as well, and last but not least, the societal influence and impact on her 'freedom of choice'. The ongoing consequence is that the question of desire for the gestational/ surrogate woman can be looked at differently if she is living in a low-income country, a country at war (as in Ukraine) or in Western society.

In this chapter, my aim is not to give a detailed overview of the different surrogacy practices, but rather to unfold the framework I have developed in the Brussels fertility center where I work. I make the hypothesis that a common ground can be found beyond the different practices that take place around the world to help us think and represent the complexity of this clinical practice.

This model embraces the different protagonists at the origin of the conception of a child with the help of a third party, which in this case can include up to five individuals. The framework that I describe in the following pages allows to explore the complex weaving and interweaving processes of desires, projections, fantasies, and stories, in all their diversity, that are at play and triggered in the various protagonists involved in the conception of an imaginary and not yet real baby. The aim of the framework is to enable the construction of a crucible/container of diverse representations resulting from a dreaming process in which the place of the imaginary baby and its various variations will nestle, hopefully allowing the psychic transformational process of symbolization to continue after the birth of the real child.

In Belgium, there is no legal frame for surrogacy, which implies it is accepted, but with the consequence that there is no legal recognition and protection for either the genetic filiation (of the intended mother) or social filiation (in the case of gay couples) of the intended parents, neither for the gestational woman. This means there is no legal recognition of a contractual agreement between the protagonists to protect the interests and security of each one and finally for the child to come. Despite the progressive augmentation of requests, the practice remains quite marginalized: in 2019 it represented 0.08 % of all cycles carried out in Belgian fertility clinics (Belrap, 2019).

Unlike in the USA, Canada, and India, amongst other countries, where the surrogate or gestational carrier can legally be paid, in our country, only the expenses in relation with ART and the pregnancy are legally authorized and are taken in charge by the intended parents. Nevertheless, such legal void has different consequences and difficulties to overcome for both parties.

One of the first consequences, and not the least, is the legal non-recognition from the beginning of the conception of the intended parental bond (genetic and symbolic) with the embryo/fetus/child and the recognition of the contractual agreements between the parties.

As a result, the surrogate mother and her husband (if she is married) are legally the child's parents (during the pregnancy and after the birth) until they legally relinquish their parental rights in favor of the intended parents, who will then have to adopt their child.

This has important consequences on a practical and administrative level, but also symbolically. Thus, the signing of the contractual documents necessary to start the reproductive procedures is the result of an agreement built up after many discussions and sealed by the weaving of a relationship based on reciprocal trust between the intended parents and the gestational candidate. This is a long process which includes the exploration of many questions, as well as the importance to include from the beginning of the process the thinking over, and then subsequently to decide, where the delivery will take place. Either in Belgium, where the gestational carrier is recognized by law "as the mother of the child" or in France (more rarely chosen) where the woman will give birth 'anonymously' to the child (*accouchement sous X*) and "abandons the child to the state's child welfare". Practically, both situations require long administrative procedures in order to legalize and recognize the filiation of the baby to the intendent parents: administrative procedures of adoption of their child either directly from the gestational woman – after she has renounced her legal filiation rights – or by the path of adopting the baby from the state's welfare. In Belgium, the intended father with a genetic filiation can legally recognize his filiation to the child before delivery, with the necessity – if the gestational woman is married – that her husband renounces during pregnancy his paternal rights.

Nevertheless, either choice will entail long administrative procedures that will continue to confront the parents with the difficulty of creating and recognizing their family, with symbolic consequences. In both cases, the symbolic process of becoming parents, linked with the recognition by the social group – with its legal frame – will be recognized *in a second phase*: after the birth of the baby. Thus, the symbolic process of passing from the status 'being the child of' to the status of 'being the parent of' needs to be recognized legally and socially in this second phase, concomitantly with the recognition of the legal filiation to their child. This temporality can be looked at as an *après-coup* and questions the symbolic impact of the societal environment, including its prejudices on the recognition of parental identity and parental functions, as well as the place given to the child (Aulagnier, 1975) by the socius, adding to the representational task of *rêverie* (Bion 1959, 1962) the need for the parents and for the child to face and process the socius' reaction.

And from the gestational woman's point of view, the non-legal recognition of her contractual engagement in the task of carrying a baby for the intended parents, questions the limits of boundaries of her protection and her rights, such as financial questions that could occur in case of medical problems during pregnancy if the intended parents refuse to pay, or in case the intended parents flee/abandon the project, and the list is non exhaustive ... a legal void where the rights of the child are also questioned! Many of these questions will be addressed during the meetings that will take place with the analyst.

The clinical frame

Having worked in a fertility center for more than a decade, I have had the opportunity to witness the broadening of the variety of the requests in the patient base population addressing themselves to a medically assisted reproduction pole. Requests for surrogacy practice have also widened, extending the field of application to different family structures in a societal climate of non-discrimination based on gender, sexual orientation, social and family situation and financial capacity (Belgium is the second most progressive country in Europe after the Netherlands, legalizing same sex marriage since June 2003, in comparison with neighboring countries).

The conception of a child by the path of surrogacy not only needs as many as five adults, but it also is a process that has medical, psycho-dynamic, and relational repercussions in the family environment of both parties, all of which must be addressed.

Practically, our center takes in family projects emanating from heterosexual couples where the woman has a medical uterine sterility (hysterectomy in case of womb cancer or due to pathological hemorrhage during childbirth, congenital sterility in the case of Rokitansky syndrome) or from homosexual men (single or in couple). We also consider more rare requests where the desire for a child is present in the woman concomitantly with a refusal of pregnancy despite the absence of medical reasons. This discrepancy between the psyche and soma – where there are neither medical nor infertility problems opposing to a pregnancy – will be questioned and explored as deeply as all other requests. In these situations, the desire to become a mother is present, but the idea of being pregnant is infiltrated with many conflictual feelings of anxiety and fear. The meetings with the analyst are an important moment to explore the preconscious and unconscious factors underlying the project.

It takes a minimum of six months to a year between the first consultations and the start of the process of procreation. This first phase consists of meeting all the participants for the conception of the child: the intended parents, the gestational woman (and her husband when married), the egg donor (for gay couples or when the intended mother is infertile) and the sperm donor (when the intended father is infertile). This first phase of the process is an important moment for the assessment of the project from medical, legal and psychological points of view.

In Belgium, it is the intended parents' responsibility to find a match with a gestational carrier. Quite often the candidate is a family member or comes from a close relationship network, and most often the relationship between the intended parents and the gestational carrier has existed for a long time, or if not, their meeting together contains an emotional load described as being very important for the future development of the project.

This first phase is characterized as a founding moment for the family project's feasibility during which a network of trusting partnerships will continue to weave or not between the intended parents and the gestational carrier and with the medical team.

Indeed, it's a period when everyone becomes aware of the impact and consequences of the complexity of the factual reality of the procedure on their daily lives, with the accompanying corollary of psychic, emotional and relational issues. Most often, it's usually during this first phase that projects are stopped either from the medical point of view (as a result of a pluri-disciplinary decision including the psycho-dynamic perspective) or from the intended parents' side or from the gestational carrier vertex. This last case has the serious consequence of putting the difficulty to find a gestational woman at the fore once again.

Building a transitional space: a third area of essential paradox

Winnicott's (1968) last writings describing an "essential paradox" at the core of his model on transitional phenomena helps us to think about the paradox encountered in the conception of a child through surrogacy. Indeed, when we think about the conception through surrogacy, it is more than a shared body for two that is at stake, it is also a time-space process in which the intended parents and the gestational woman will be involved together both in external reality in the conception and giving birth to a child, *and* in a shared subjective experience containing all the corollaries linked with intra and intersubjective psychic reality processes. It is a lifelong ongoing process that will continue after the birth of the child, where the relational patterns of the intended parents with the gestational woman (and her family) will often continue to weave; the gestational woman (and her family) being often part of the enlarged family network.

Thus, conceptualizing the different encounters that will take place with the participants of the project as a third area is a model that allows different functions to be highlighted. Considering and representing this time-space moment taking place in an intermediate area including "the essential paradox which has to do with living experience and is neither dream nor object-relating" (Winnicott, 1968, p. 204) opens up a space, a transitional area, with its fundamental function in the processes of symbolization and in the construction of the subjectivity for the future child to come. It is in this space, in the course of an ongoing process, that the symbolic function at play from the origin of the family project will be put to work in the complex task of an interweaving working process by both parties during meetings with the intended parents and the gestational carrier (and her husband, if she is married).

This model of framework also functions as a container for the exploration of a vast array of questions, narratives, projections and fantasies, including the sensorial and emotional climate linked to the ongoing discussions.

Practically, it is during this phase that conceptual questions are discussed and explored thoroughly during the alternating meetings with the intended parents and with the gestational carrier (and her husband).

Thus, the building of the frame and the follow-up sessions are specific to each process. In some cases, it eventually includes the necessity of meeting different family members, either of the intended parents or of the gestational woman.

During this first period, the building of a transitional area is fostered by the opening, exploration and discussion of many topics and questions such as the many "what ifs", "what would you decide?", "who will decide?", "who will be included in the decision taking?", "what are the limitations/boundaries in the implication in the project?", "when to stop?".

The analyst's function, while accompanying both parties to explore this vast array of questions with a foundation in reality, is to address them as 'imaginary' scenarios involving the intended parents, the gestational woman (and her family), or the not-yet-real baby, placing the imaginary baby at the core.

In these scenarios, the imaginary baby 'not yet real' is dreamt with the specificity of being a baby that will be carried in the mind of the intended parents and in the body and psyche of the gestational woman. An imaginary baby also needs to be thought not only in the intended parents' family network, but also with its impact in the relational network of the gestational woman's family.

Some examples to be thought, talked and imagined: "what will happen to the not yet born baby during the pregnancy in the eventuality of separation/death of the intended parents?"; "what can one think in the case of an embryo/baby abnormality diagnosed during the pregnancy? Who decides how to proceed?"; "Who will decide of a medical interruption of pregnancy?"; "What are the limitations for the gestational woman to accept to continue the pregnancy if a malformation is diagnosed? And for the intended parents?"; "What relationship do the intended parents imagine/wish for between the child and the gestational woman (and her family)?"; "How does the gestational woman imagine the pregnancy of a child that she hasn't desired, and what kind of relationship does she imagine having with the baby during pregnancy and after having given birth?"; "What if the gestational woman encounters health problems during pregnancy? Or her husband or their children?"; "Has the gestational woman (and her husband) thought of the risks of pregnancy and eventual death?";"Has this risk been thought about by the intended parents?"; "Where will the birth take place?"; "How does the gestational woman imagine her pregnancy and relationship with the embryo/baby?"; "Does she imagine herself talking to the baby, how to name a baby that is not hers?", "How will her children name the baby, and represent their relationship, with a baby growing in their mother's womb and with no kinship to them?" And this list is not exhaustive. Questions will continue to emerge progressively as the imaginary family network of relationship weaves and extends itself to include a larger group of family members.

There are many practical questions that are usually not thought about before conception in a classical way, that imperatively need to be discussed and are part of the building of the contractual agreement based on trust.

The ongoing dialogue that continues between the meetings will hopefully help the weaving of narratives containing representations of the family network in construction and the consolidation of a shared space where the place of the baby is elaborated. These scenarios are taken up subsequently with the analyst, allowing the exploration of subjective imaginary scenarios that continues to foster other thoughts not yet thought, which results in the creation of an interweaving intersubjective area, metaphorically a container – a nest – for the imaginary baby to come, at the core of the psychic process of becoming parents.

The analyst placing herself at the crossroads of the transitional area, fostering these questions, on a conceptual and subjective mode, also opens for the possibility to "play with ideas" (Winnicott, 1971), and helps to maintain/create a field of reflection and of *rêverie*, infiltrated by the implication of wishes and desires in an area where phantasmatic scenarios have all their place to playfully oscillate between internal and external reality. An area that comes before objectivity and perceptibility of a real baby, where the borders of bodily intimacy, sexual fantasies and boundaries weave and build through different narratives, paving the path for the reproduction process to take place in a 'shared space' between the gestational woman and the intended parents.

This allows from the intended parents' point of view the development of the parental *rêverie*, essential for attachment and bonding to a child and for the building of parental identity, but with the *essential paradox* of taking place in another body-mind environment, the one of the gestational carrier. This model also allows for the gestational woman (and her family environment) to explore the same questions, narratives, with its specific projections, fantasies, sensorial and bodily experiences occurring during the process, with the specificity of accepting to carry a baby which is part of someone else's parental desire. Indeed, for the gestational carrier, offering her body to carry and give birth to a child, the conception of 'a shared space', is implicit and contains the woman's unconscious incentives underlying her desire to take part in the creation of a family through surrogacy.

The transitional area, quoting Winnicott's thought on the essential paradox published in the "Tailpiece" from *Playing and Reality* (1971, p. 151), where "at the theoretical beginning a baby can be said to live in a subjective or conceptual world. The change from the primary state to one in which objective perception is possible is not only a matter of inherent or inherited growth process; it needs in addition a minimum environment. It belongs to the whole vast theme of the individual travelling from dependence towards independence", which is an area mirroring reflective and reflexive exchanges that will emerge, fostering images, fantasies and representations of the conception of a baby with 'many-others'. This essential paradox is intrinsic to surrogacy, where a gap between conception and perception is present since the origin – a caesura (Bion, [1977] 2011) triggering the capacity of dreaming for both the intended parents and the gestational carrier at the origin of the baby's life.

Discussions progressively deepen in content, where the imaginary baby's representations and his/her place in the surrogacy family matrix, as well as the baby's place in the gestational woman's psyche and family matrix are omnipresent.

These meetings also trigger the individual capacity to negotiate with one's own capacity of metabolization of phantasmatic scenarios linked to the baby-making with a birth-other from a biological point of view. It is not rare that phantasmatic scenarios with a sexual connotation emerge underlying questions concerning the conception of the embryo or while talking about the building of a zone of intimacy between the two parties with a common shared space. Questions such as "who will assist at the consultation with the gynecologist?"; or "where will the intended parents be while the transfer of the embryo takes place? or during delivery?" convey psycho-sexual reverberations triggering phantasmatic representations about the origin of life. Some phantasmatic scenarios can also be conveyed by other family members, such as for example from an eight-year-old child of the gestational candidate asking his mother if "she would have to have sex with Paul or with Keith to make their baby?"

This is an ongoing life process that each participant in the project will be confronted with, forcing everyone to grapple with the construction of the foundations for the family matrix. This process includes keeping in mind the complex developmental task the birth-other child born through surrogacy has to progressively represent and understand his family matrix pattern of relationship, including the different birth-others, and to elaborate in an ongoing process the "multiple circulating narratives" (Corbert, 2017) related to his or her existence before, during and after conception.

Francis shares his feeling during a session with his husband at a moment preceding the beginning of the reproduction process. Describing how much he felt relieved to finally start the procedure but at the same time having a weird feeling when he thinks and becomes aware of what is opening up; and he puts it as follows: to be at the threshold of becoming father of their baby, which will be carried by Anna who will have no genetic link with the baby, but who will at the same time be the one who will have so much intimacy with the baby .... What a complex task to integrate!

Underlying this narrative, a vast array of condensed elements can be found and for some will continue to unfold and transform during the meetings, such as fantasies of the primal scene mixed with infantile sexual scenarios ("to be at the threshold of becoming father ... carried by Anna who will have no genetic link.... What a complex task to integrate!") or maternal representations mixed with a hint of rivalry and of gratitude ("Anna ... who will at the same time be the one who will have so much intimacy with the baby ...").

Francis' thoughts also reflect the conflicting and paradoxical position of being grateful to Anna for agreeing to carry their baby, while at the same time having to deal with ambivalent emotions infiltrated by the guilt of worrying about the bond that will develop between Anna and the baby.

These conflicting feelings and thoughts were mixed with the relief of Anna's trust and emotional care of the baby during pregnancy, as was often discussed during the long process leading up to this long-awaited moment!

Francis' question also opens the field of the importance the gestational woman has on the origins of the psychic life of the baby and on what psycho-analysis refers to as the proto-mental-traces.

Nevertheless, this frame can also fail. Indeed, meeting the analyst is a moment characterized by the opening and sharing the family project with a third, in a new space: the fertility center. The emotional and symbolic impact of triangulation with the analyst with whom different relational patterns will be explored is crucial. Indeed, the co-construction process of talking, sharing thoughts and scenarios has usually already started privately between the intended parents and the gestational carrier (and her husband, and eventually with their children) before addressing their request to the fertility center. In some circumstances, this triangulation with its inherent consequence of open-ing a transitional area will not take place, often bringing the project to an end.

Clinical vignette

This is what happened at the end of a few meetings with Timothy and John, who came to our fertility center asking help for the surrogacy family project they had built and weaved with Sue, the gestational carrier candidate, and her wife Jane, in the last six months.

At our first meeting, Timothy took a leading position being quite direct in sharing with me his discomfort and irritation about the aim of our meetings, "not being in the need to share their concerns", as he put it out clearly, "as they (meaning both couples) had taken a lot of time to build a relationship of trust which allowed them to talk about and go through different issues together". Timothy could nevertheless understand the importance of talking about the complexity of surrogacy conception in general, but found that it didn't concern "their personal project". John sat back listening in silence and seemed quite worried. After a while, he tried to excuse Timothy's irritation, attributing it to the many tensions and difficulties they had already gone through since they first desired to build a family together and become parents. This was an impor-tant and crucial moment: I could sense the intensity of contained pain mixed with anger that both Timothy and John tried to protect themselves from, put-ting me in the position 'of another obstacle to pass' and projecting on the analyst their fear of being stopped 'again'.

A moment where the re-actualization of past failures that have paved their project up to now were inevitably brought to surface and projected in the future.

This pivotal moment, opening the possibility to revisit the past story – with its inherent pains, tensions and fantasies – is only possible if an encounter where triangulation can be established can take place. With Timothy and John, each encounter was infiltrated with an atmosphere of suspicion and distrust and the same defensive pattern was put forward, defeating all my attempts to build a collaboration. Of course, I gathered some information about their life and background, but all were shared on a factual mode, not giving me any access to explore with them, for example, the questions and issues they had discussed with Sue and Jane that for them built their contractual agreement. Leaving me with no representations of the family network they had imagined in their couple, nor with Sue nor Jane, nor about their agreements about the pregnancy with its inherent risks. Every attempt from my side was received as an attack: it was as if I was facing a rock, with the consequence of intensifying the defenses. Transferentially, I was put at the place of an intruder with whom a battle had to take place in order to protect what Timothy called "the privacy of their family project with the help of Sue". I didn't have the occasion to have information about the place of the child in the family network Timothy, John, Sue and Jane thought about, as the sessions were put to an end at Timothy's request.

Despite the non-encounter and the failure of opening and triangulation of the family project with the analyst, this example also unveils the complex and intense emotional turmoil with corollary defense mechanisms that are met within the fertility clinic and the impact of the complex and painful path of 'birth-other' family construction has on the subject.

The failure of the creation of a transitional area didn't allow the opening of their project to a third, with the consequence that the triangulation, 'to see, to look, to be seen' – represented here by the analyst – was perceived as too dangerous for Timothy and John. In this case, the function of assessment endorsed by the analyst was impossible to work through, and to transform in a representational process: the analyst being perceived in a schizo-paranoid position and endorsing all the painful and unresolved traumatic events of the past, leaving open the field of the underlying unconscious, relational, traumatic, transgenerational, cultural reasons at stake.

Some thoughts from the woman's gestational vertex

Many questions arise concerning the conscious and unconscious incentives grounding the woman's desire to engage herself – comprising all the consequences for her family environment – to undertake such a complex path, including taking the risk of putting one's life in danger during the process of pregnancy, until birth. This is a project where the assessment of the place of the imaginary baby – with its narcissistic and objectal oscillations – has an important place, to talk about a baby 'as a subject-to-be', but who will grow in her body and will interact with her by sensory-motor pathways.

In Belgium, due to the absence of legal frame, the gestational woman is often related to one of the intended parents (cousin, sister-in-law, close friend) or is found through close relationship (a friend of an aunt, a friend of a close friend). The two parties have often met before and this encounter is often described by the gestational candidate as an intense emotional moment. This emotional factor is an important element at the origin of the engagement and consent of the gestational woman in the project, described as one of the founding pillars for the weaving and strengthening of the relationship of trust. We could think of this moment as an encounter that mobilizes intense (sometimes massive) inter-psychic processes and at the same time conveys its underlying conscious and unconscious motivations.

Very often the desire of helping another woman or man to become a parent is present long before the idea of surrogacy. The conscious motivations vary and are grounded on singular unconscious incentives that are not easy to reveal, as the setting of meetings with gestational candidates is not a psychoanalysis. But some clues of unconscious incentives can be found in the narratives that unfold during the evolving meetings. For example, during the meetings, Myriam, the gestational woman for Helen and Robert, shared her memory of having thought "even before she became a mother" that one day she would also help others (women or men) to become parents of a child. This desire Myriam linked with her child memory of "always wanting to repair what doesn't work". Or while meeting June, gestational candidate for her brother-in-law (brother of her husband), who described how painful it was for her to witness the difficulty her brother-in-law faced with his husband in their wish to become parents, which played a role in the decision she took to first talk with them and offer herself to become their gestational carrier. Or at the first meeting with Elsa, sharing with me with great emphasis her willingness to become the surrogate for Ted and John's project of having a child: "Since I was young, I always wanted to help in one way or another somebody that couldn't have children. Then, since I became a mother and experienced pregnancy so easily, I imagined I could also do the same for someone who couldn't .... and I saw a program on surrogacy and that's how I first started to think about the idea of being a surrogate mother ... and of offering to someone my capacity of bearing a child..."

The conscious motivations are often described as altruistic: 'to help the other in difficulty', a position where the identification with 'the pain of not being able to' is a driving force. Nevertheless, unconscious motivations, the unseen scenarios, are also part of the process and eventually these will appear during the time-space created for the meetings that take place in the fertility center, before and after conception. Scenarios surface that show the unconscious search for a reward and subjective recognition from the other, or fantasies of reparation of transgenerational figures, or an unfulfilled process of mourning.

Later, Elsa expressed that she could no longer endure the fertility process and the feeling of failure after the two transfer essays which led to the loss of two embryos and decided that she should stop the procedure and not start another cycle. She felt sad for John and Ted's sadness, struggling not to feel guilty of not having been able to fulfill her engagement, but her own sadness was too intense, a sorrow that she hadn't felt when she miscarried many years ago. She suddenly realized the pain she felt now wasn't only about the miscarriage of John and Ted's embryo, but it was also about the mourning of her past experience of miscarriage that only now she had started feeling.

From the analyst's vertex: the counter-transferential process

In this model, the analyst takes part in the process since the first consultation at the fertility center and also in the pluri-disciplinary decision of accepting the surrogate project or not. It is a position that can be discussed as it implies taking into account the transferential impact (positive and negative) and the consequences of this position for every subject, with all its conscious and unconscious repercussions.

The clear communication of the working frame is a very important moment and implies taking time to clearly explain the forthcoming procedure, consisting on alternating meetings with each party in a frame that also adapts itself according to the forthcoming necessities. The analyst introduces her function as a mediator in order to explore the project both parties have shared, together with its inherent limitations. The analyst will also explain that during the meeting process, different issues and their adjacent scenarios will be explored in order to encourage dialogue, questions and representations between each participant.

From a psychoanalytical point of view, the analyst's mediator function is to be understood as a function of a malleable mediating object, where the analyst not only guarantees the frame containing a transitional area, but also has a catalyzer function for symbolization. By adopting a position of receptivity and offering oneself as a malleable object (Milner 1952, Roussillon, 1988, 2015), the analyst helps the weaving of a fabric of narratives, scenarios, fantasies, that also implies the differentiation of non-shared areas with their limiting envelopes and frontiers.

There is no doubt that the relationship of dependence on the gestational carrier often inhibits the intended parents, who adopt a more passive position, waiting for the gestational carrier to "authorize" them to take part in the process (as for example the medical exams inherent to the conception of their child or later during pregnancy). The creation of shared and non-shared spaces gradually takes shape during the process, and this experience will enable new developments and transformations once the process is underway.

The analyst's listening of the narratives including the fantasies and defense mechanisms helps to maintain/create a field of reflection and of *rêverie* bringing together the fantasies of each participant in a family *rêverie* with a particular focus on what is kept silent. The analyst's negative capacity of listening, including the sensorial proto-mental aspects, plays a part on the counter-transferential work of *rêverie*. The analyst accepts endorsing projections and fantasies and fostering the dreaming function of each party offering an environment sufficiently malleable, a transitional area that participates in the constitution of the premises of a nest for the child to come.

The ongoing counter-transferential work, as well as the ethical stance of the "responsibility for the other" (Lévinas, 1982), is part of the process, mirroring the incessant weaving work put in motion from the first meeting with all the partners, engaging since the origin in the building of a surrogate family.

Some open questions from the child's vertex

Undoubtedly the child developmental outcome includes the processing of his/her family romance and origin from surrogacy. It is a delicate interweaving process of intrapsychic and intersubjective factors allowing representations, fantasies, narratives of relationships with the caretakers and birth-others actors of his/her life, which hopefully allows to develop his/her sense of Self and of the Other.

Nevertheless, many questions remain open about the embodied traces of the intra-uterine life of the fetus/baby – or proto-representations in a Bionian perspective –, intimately linked and in a reflective dialectic mode of support to the gestational environment and the question of the emergence of thought. As unfolds in Maiello's (2000) work on the role of "sound object" of the mother's voice having a role in the foundation of the psyche and its role in proto-mental representation of presence-absence.

What will be the impact for the baby when after birth he/she is given to his/her parents by the gestational woman? A moment of sensorial transition from one environment to another where the dreaming and alpha capacity of the parents is crucial.

Many questions englobing psychological, biological and relational domains remain open to explore in the future. These issues are to be closely linked with the ongoing psychic development of the sense of self and identity, without omitting to link the impact of the social environment and cultural norms and prejudices on the children's development.

Conclusion

The conception of a child with the help of ART is nowadays practiced in many parts of the world. Since its first steps, it has allowed many adults to become parents and many children to be born with or without gamete donation. It is nowadays a contemporary clinical practice closely linked to biomedical progress, technology and socio-cultural trends allowing the creation of new family configurations. It is a specific evolving clinical practice arousing new questions to be thought, closely linked to ethics and to the specific legal frame of each country where ART is practiced, putting our psychoanalytical clinical and theoretical models to the test.

Building a family through surrogacy is a complex route that needs to bring together up to five adults for the conception of a child with the help of ART. Meeting the different protagonists in the fertility center allows to open a time-space framework putting everyone at work in an anticipatory way, thinking and talking about 'the best scenarios', as well as 'the worst scenarios' that can happen in the process of reproduction and during pregnancy. It is an occasion to foster the elaboration of narratives that help to represent and to maintain in tension the place of the imaginary child at the center of the crossroads of everyone taking part of the project.

Fostering narratives and storytelling is a very important function during these encounters. This psychic capacity is anchored at the core of the imaginary dreaming creativity of each adult and plays an important role in the early parent-infant relationship, an object relational setting within which the infant's early experience of sense of self will take place and constitutes part of the unthought known (Bollas, 1987). We can assume that facilitating an ongoing process of narratives and storytelling from the origin helps the future parents to transmit to the child the knowledge of the different protagonists of his existence and the building of a family story.

Nevertheless, the uncertainty of how the child will negotiate during his/her psycho-developmental process the complex relational network at the origin of his/her existence will remain. As well as the various accompanying and evolving fantasy scenarios, with their specific conscious and unconscious aspects, that the child will experience in the course of his/her development and will have to deal with, without forgetting to take into account the not-inconsiderable impact of cultural norms and prejudices on unconventional families that are met in different parts of the world.

References

Aulagnier-Castoriadis, P. (1975). *La violence de l'interprétation*. Presses Universitaires de France.

Bion, W.R. (1959). Attacks on linking. *International Journal of Psychoanalysis*, 40: 308–315.

Bion, W.R. (1962). A theory of thinking. *International Journal of Psychoanalysis*, 43: 306–310.

Bion, W.R. ([1977] 2011). *Two papers: "The grid" and "Caesura"*. Karnac.

Bollas, C. (1987). *The shadow of the object*. Free Association Press.

Corbert, K. (2017). Nontraditional family romance. *The Psychoanalytic Quarterly* 70: 683–711. DOI: 10.1002/j.2167-4086.2001.tb00613.x

College of Physicians of Reproductive Medicine (2019). *IVF Report*. Available online in https://www.belrap.be/Documents/Reports/Global/FinalReport_IVF19_28OCT21.pdf

Ehrensaft, D. (2000). Alternatives to the stork fatherhood fantasies in donor insemination families. *Studies in Gender and Sexuality*, 1: 371–397. DOI:10.1080/15240650109349165

Ehrensaft, D. (2005). *Mommies, daddies, donors, surrogates*. Guilford.

Ehrensaft, D. (2008). When baby makes three or four or more. *Psychoanalytic Study of the Child*, 63: 3–23. DOI: 10.1080/00797308.2008.11800797

Lévinas, E. (1982). *Éthique et infini. Dialogues avec Philippe Nemo*. Fayard.

Maiello, S. (2000). Trames sonores et rythmiques primordiales: Reminiscences auditives dans le travail psychanalytique. *Journal de la psychanalyse de l'enfant*, 26: 77–103.

Milner, M. (1952). Aspects of symbolism in comprehension of the not-self. *International Journal of Psychoanalysis*, 33: 181–194.

Roussillon, R. (1988). Le medium malléable, la représentation de la représentation et la pulsion d'emprise. *Revue Belge de Psychanalyse*, 13: 71–87.

Roussillon, R. (2015). An introduction to the work on primary symbolization. *International Journal of Psychoanalysis*, 96: 583–594.

Winnicott, D. (1968). Playing and culture. In *Psychoanalytic Explorations* (pp. 203–206). Harvard University Press.

Winnicott, D. (1971). *Playing and Reality*. Tavistock.

Index

www.ingramcontent.com/pod-product-compliance
Ingram Content Group UK Ltd.
Pitfield, Milton Keynes, MK11 3LW, UK
UKHW022351040225
454686UK00011B/50